It's Not About The Cheesecake

Sulana Perelman

It's Not About The Cheesecake
www.It'sNotAboutTheCheesecake.com
Copyright © 2017 by Sulana Perelman

Limits of Liability and Disclaimer of Warranty

Publisher
10-10-10 Publishing
Markham, ON
Canada

Printed in the United States of America
ISBN: 978-1-77277-124-4

Contents

Acknowledgements

I am very blessed to have support and guidance from many wonderful people to whom I want to express my sincere gratitude:

To my partner Marco, who goes along with my crazy ideas, supports me in everything I do, and tells me that I am special every single day.

To my children Sam and Bayla, who bring light, purpose, and love into my life.

To my parents, Edward and Mila, who have always been a prime example of love, family, and kindness.

To my best friend, Laura, who has listened, consoled, laughed, and celebrated with me for over 30 years.

To Raymond Aaron for his passion for life and helping make the impossible, possible.

To Cara Witvoet, my Personal Book Architect, for her positivity, assistance, and guidance.

To Lisa Browning, my Editor, for her feedback and expertise.

Testimonials

"Just imagine hearing compliments about the way you look and how good that would make you feel. Sulana's book "It's Not About The Cheesecake" is not only innovative, informative and thought-provoking, it puts you in the driver's seat of your life, allowing you to create real and sustainable change!"

Michael E. Moore, TMNLP, MTLT, TMCHt, Certified Fitness Trainer

"Most weight loss books only deal with meal plans and exercise regimes. Sulana will help you transform your thinking about dieting, and guide you to the underlying reasons why you continue to struggle with weight and what you can do about it."

Lennie Iskender, Registered Dietitian

"Sulana's book, "It's Not About The Cheesecake," really speaks to women who have been battling with their weight. Her very simple and practical tools will help you uncover your deeper limiting issues and the action steps to take to move forward."

Jacqueline Betterton, TV Host and Producer

Foreword

If you are fed up with yo-yo dieting and emotional eating, and are ready to do something different, something that will work, *It's Not About The Cheesecake* is the book you have to read.

Sulana has counselled women with weight issues for almost 20 years. After seeing one client after another not able to maintain their weight loss goals, she made it her mission to find out what works, and share her knowledge with you.

You may have been blaming yourself for lacking willpower, coming up short in your dieting efforts, or feeling like a failure. You will finally grasp why the next "perfect" diet will set you up for disappointment, and what you absolutely must know and do in order to be successful.

Written in a way that grabs your attention from page one, reading *It's Not About The Cheesecake* will make you will feel like you are chatting with Sulana over coffee. Sulana is open and direct, and shares her personal struggles with weight and how she was able to get control over her eating. You will learn techniques that have worked for Sulana and her clients, and you will feel empowered and excited to start your personal journey to success.

Raymond Aaron
New York Times Bestselling Author

Introduction

Time To Get Off The Hamster Wheel To Nowhere

Your next diet won't work. Go ahead, try it, and see what happens. Deep down you probably already know that, don't you?

As a Registered Dietitian, I refuse to put you on a diet. For your own good. Diets don't work and they will never work for you. Ever. I know what you may be thinking: "Wow, isn't this a cheerful book I'm about to read and, by the way, isn't the word 'DIET' actually in your professional title? Isn't that the reason to see a Dietitian in the first place? To. Go. On. A. Diet?" Well, I can appreciate your concern. Let me explain.

I've been a practicing Registered Dietitian for over 18 years. If you would have come to my office 5 years ago and told me you wanted to lose weight, I would have put you on a diet. Or, as we say in the profession, a "healthy eating plan." We would have discussed your lifestyle, eating habits, and physical activity, and I would have then simply provided you with a meal plan to follow for the rest of your life. Easy peasy. Two weeks later, we would meet again; you would proudly get weighed and the results would show a loss of a few pounds. It's working!!! So we would chat some more and I would give you more advice and recommendations, and maybe some recipes, and send you on your way. This would continue for a few more visits, of course. You would be feeling better, have more energy, be motivated, and perhaps you would have even decided to add physical activity into your daily regime and be well on your way to fitting into that dress hanging in the back of your closet! Then, there is the fifth visit. You come in feeling distraught. You tell me you almost cancelled the visit. You were "bad" and didn't follow your healthy eating plan. You had a birthday party in your home and you ate a big piece of cake that evening (It was double chocolate with gooey caramel sauce and whipped cream with cherries on top!), and then you ate 3 pieces of the cake for breakfast the next day. And, to make matters worse, you ordered take-out for dinner that night and for dinner the day after. During your visit with me, the scale reveals that you have gained 3 pounds since our last appointment. You feel so disappointed. You vow to get back on track, back to the plan that was working. You've got it all under control. The next visit, the scale shows another 2 pounds of weight gain. You admit to be back to snacking in the evening after the kids go to bed. You are mad at yourself and say that you know what you have to do to get back on track. You remember how "good" you were before at following the recommendations. All you have to do is just go back to what you were doing before. A few days before the next visit, you call me to tell me that you need to cancel and will call later to rebook. You don't reschedule.

Does this scenario sound familiar? It's familiar to me because I'd see it repeat itself with many of my clients who came to see me for weight loss. I felt that I could almost predict when their weight loss would halt and the weight regain would begin. I felt at a loss! I could see how excited they were to embark on a new healthy plan at our first meeting. They wanted to succeed so desperately! They were truly tired of being overweight and not being able to feel good about themselves. I was ecstatic to bestow all my knowledge in nutrition that could help them achieve their weight goals. I would be there to make sure they were eating enough to meet their nutritional and caloric requirements that would not leave them hungry; I was there to provide them with delicious and easy recipes so that meal preparation was simple; I was there to show them the benefits of exercise; I was there to encourage them every step of the way. Yet all of this knowledge and support did not help them to continue on their healthy journey for the long term.

Some of the clients that I counselled lost a small amount of weight (5 or 10 pounds), while others were able to lose a significant amount of weight (20 pounds, 30 pounds, 60 pounds). Maintaining that weight loss was the hurdle that many could not overcome. You would think that this would be the easier part—the maintenance. But that ended up being the hardest part. The almost impossible part. All of this knowledge and information that I offered my clients, and giving them the impression that it was about willpower, failed them in their attempts at losing weight. I knew my clients truly wanted to be successful at their weight loss efforts. I was an empathetic practitioner with a lot of knowledge and experience, and I was eager to share with them what I had learned, but I realized that teaching clients about healthy eating and nutrition and exercise was just not enough.

The statistics ARE stacked against dieters. The majority of dieters regain the weight they lose, and then some. I didn't realize it at the time, but I was trying to solve my clients' weight issues completely the wrong way. I was focusing on how much and what they ate, and the amount of exercise they included in the week. I was only looking at the surface of their weight issues, not knowing that successfully getting rid of the weight and keeping it off is not about the perfect diet and the best meal plan.

> *Focusing only on the surface issues of being overweight will not result in lasting success.*

Even back then, I realized that the attainment and maintenance of weight loss went much deeper than just "eating healthy and exercising." My clients were not *bad*, or *failures*, or other words they called themselves. They honestly wanted to lose the weight and have a healthy body and lifestyle, and be free of the food obsession, but they could not sustain it. Not long term. In my gut, I knew that there must be more to it than knowing the correct portion size of your chicken breast. Why? Because it's not about the food!

I could completely relate to my clients and their weight struggles. I was a closet yo-yo dieter for many years. My first dieting attempt began when I was 11 years of age and found one of my mother's diet books. It was around that time that I hit puberty and was getting "chubby." I remember standing in front of the mirror with my best friend as we discussed our bodies from head to toe and everything that was wrong with us. Diets played a big part in my life growing up. It was "the thing" to do. Overate at a dinner party? Next day, start a diet. Ate too many desserts? Dieting is the answer! This was common dinner conversation. I would only give myself permission to reach for a piece of cake because I knew that the next day, I would start atoning for my sins by dieting. This ended up becoming my way of life: binge eat and gain weight, followed by crash diet to lose weight.

My yo-yo dieting continued past my teens and into my twenties and thirties. It's not difficult to understand why I chose this profession. I thought that I could help others and hopefully help myself. I would sit and listen to my clients complain that they were not able to stick to their diets and I could completely relate. Here I was teaching clients about weight loss, and I could not get a hold of my own weight issues. It's like a doctor who smokes, telling his patients about the perils of smoking. I could not admit this to anyone. I thought I was doing a great job at hiding my weight struggles, of course, because it was the same 10–15 pounds that I lost and regained. It wasn't completely unnoticeable but, with the right wardrobe modifications, I thought I was doing a good job at concealing it. Losing weight equaled tighter clothes; regaining weight equaled loose and flowy blouses. I felt like a fraud. And a hypocrite.

Why am I sharing all this with you? I want you to know that I've been there. I've struggled with dieting and beat myself up for my lack of willpower. There were days when my "fat pants" were tight and I didn't want to leave the house and face the world. There were nights where I promised myself that the next day would be a new beginning. I would finally lose the weight for good. So I completely know where you are coming from. I understand your struggles. I get your disappointments. I feel your pain.

I would still be in this yo-yo cycle of unhappiness had I not been fortunate to finally figure out what works, and this is what I want to share with you. I want you to be able to break free from the dieting nonsense! I want you to wake up in the morning and be able to face the day and not have every thought be about food. I want you to love yourself and know that you are worthy of a great life. I want to share with you what will work and what you can do to finally be successful. I have been fortunate to learn about methods that changed my life and my clients' lives as well. Focusing on food and exercise, and only food and exercise, to lose weight, will only work for a small percentage of people long term. For most of the people who want to get rid of the excess weight, knowing how to eat healthy and exercise is not enough. Imagine that, I was doing my clients a disservice. I was setting them up for failure (unintentionally, of course). Me! An educated professional with a Master's Degree in Nutrition!

I will share with you in this book why the next "diet" is not your answer to losing weight. You will never have to go on another diet again. You will never have to admit that you "failed" with the latest meal plan. Why? Because I know how it feels. I know how it is to have to spend most of your waking hours thinking about food or about the fact that you can't have food. Denying your body's natural urges. Succumbing into cravings and feeling completely out of control. Always being at two extremes: restricting or overeating. Feeling motivated or depressed; feeling hungry or so full you are in pain. When you are unhappy with how you look, and you feel out of control, it not only affects you, it affects everything you do. It's time to get off that hamster wheel that keeps you going in circles and start moving toward your magnificent potential!

Chapter 1

Understanding What It's All About

Monday Means Diet

Monday should be renamed as "Start Your New Diet" day. Isn't that the day most people begin a new diet? Sunday nights are when plans are made for how the coming week will be the week of willpower. By Sunday night, you are so fed up with the lack of control you have had with your eating, you are ready to start your new plan.

So, on Sunday night you start listing all of the things you will do:

1. Wake up at 5:30 am and go for a jog, even if it kills you.

2. Go grocery shopping and only buy the *allowed* food for your meals.

3. Skip breakfast or have coffee only; no sense in packing in the calories early on.

4. Pack a healthy lunch of salad, salad, and more salad.

5. Come home and have a small size chicken breast and salad (with no dressing).

6. Tell yourself you enjoy the hunger pangs you are feeling because that means the diet is "working."

7. Avoid the drive-thru in the morning where the freshest, yummiest, blueberry muffins are sold.

8. Have your lunch in the office so that you are not tempted by any yummies your colleagues may have brought.

9. Use your willpower to not eat the foods at dinner you prepared for the rest of the family.

10. Avoid the bag of chips, cookies, and ice-cream that are calling your name after the kids are in bed.

You are all set and ready to go!

You make it through the morning with your stomach grumbling, your lunch leaves you unsatisfied and, by dinner, you are so hungry you can eat 3 meals. Nevertheless, you make it through the day, go to bed hungry, but at the same time pleased with yourself that you have made it without "being bad." As you fall asleep, you are already imagining how you will look with 40 less pounds, and all the compliments you will get from your friends and family.

Day two continues much the same way. You are motivated! You feel you are already seeing less puffiness in your face. This is simple! And so it continues like this for 1 week or 2. You are seeing results. You are constantly hungry, but you tell yourself it is worth it! And then you get invited to a restaurant for a friend's birthday. "That's ok," you think. You plan in your head all the healthy options you will choose for the dinner (salad with dressing on the side; broiled fish; vegetables with no butter; skip the dessert). You get to the restaurant and the first item that is brought to the table is hot slices of baked bread with butter on the side. You try not to look at them, but it's like they are calling out to you—"Eat me…. eat me." "Just one slice," you say to yourself. Oh, it tastes good. You begin to recall how much you've deprived yourself the last 2 weeks. You have been so good! What's one slice going to do? Doesn't mean all is lost. It's ONE slice! You savour it. I mean, who knows when you'll have a chance to eat this again. You are on a diet after all. And then, almost without thinking, you grab the second slice. And then the third. When the waitress comes to take your order, you ask for fish and chips. Once the meal arrives, it's so good, you wolf it down without even tasting it. You figure, you've already blown the diet with the bread, you might as well enjoy it. You deserve it! What's one cheat meal anyway, in the grand scheme of things! Dinner is followed by dessert. An ooey-gooey, double chocolate brownie with fudge sauce and whipped cream. YUM. You are full—more than full—you are feeling uncomfortably stuffed. But you will not leave a morsel of brownie on your plate. You will never have this brownie again. You are on a diet!

On the drive back home, you are overcome with guilt. Guilt and judgment. Aside from your stomach hurting you because you ate too much, you are berating yourself for what just happened. What happened to all of your preplanning? "If only I would have stayed away from the bread and ordered the broiled fish. What's wrong with me? Why am I so weak? How come my friend Joanie always eats dessert and doesn't gain an ounce? Why wasn't I born with a better metabolism! I have no self-control; I am so horrible; I don't even deserve to be thin." You are so upset with yourself when you get back home, you grab a stale bag of chips from the cupboard and eat the whole bag standing by the kitchen counter. "Tomorrow," you vow. "Tomorrow, I will only eat vegetables." But the next day, as you get to work, somebody brings in a box of freshly baked donuts and muffins. You decide to have one. After all, you haven't had a donut in weeks! You'll restart your diet plan tomorrow. Well, maybe not tomorrow because you have to work late and you always order pizza when you are working late. You will need your comfort food when you have pressure at work. But definitely soon. Very, very soon. Maybe next Monday…

What do you see when you get on the scale 3 weeks later? All of the weight has come back on. Plus an added bonus of 5 pounds. You can't believe it. This is horrible. "How could I have let this happen? I am such a failure," you think. You decide you need to go on a new diet that will work. One that will take the weight off fast. Didn't you hear about Megan at work who is doing a cleanse that promises to take off 7 pounds in 1 week? Now that is amazing. You decide to speak to her at work to get all the information.

Next thing you know, you are at the store buying the juices and pills and powders and whatever else you need to "cleanse your body" (by the way, that's what your liver, kidney and skin is for, to get rid of wastes and toxins from your body). The next day, you make the morning drink and have to hold your nose to get it down, it is so gross. By lunch, you are hungry, grumpy, and are doing everything not to focus on food. You are feeling miserable. On your way back home, you stop by a fast food place and order the combo dinner with the extra-large fries and drink. "Failure," you say, as you wolf down the meal.

I can run this scenario with my eyes closed. I was always either in a losing or gaining mentality. Either severely restricting what I ate and munching on carrots and celery, counting every calorie I put into my mouth, or stopping by a bakery on my way home and buying 3 éclairs to eat as I made my way home. I would then have to hide the empty bakery package so nobody knew my shame. At the restaurant, I would either be ordering fish and steamed vegetables, or eating bread with butter, cheesy pasta, and dessert. I knew about balanced eating, everything in moderation, etc., etc., etc. I could have written a book about eating for health and energy, with a ton of strategies for weight loss. The problem was not with my knowledge. The problem was sustaining any of it long term.

You may wonder why I didn't just take my own advice and eat healthier, without severe restrictions which ultimately leads to bingeing and overeating. Well, let me tell you, even when I was following a healthy, balanced way of eating, all I could focus on was the food. It was all I could think of: when my next meal would be; what my next meal would be; how many calories I had consumed already; writing down every morsel of food I ate; and on and on. Eventually, even this healthy plan began to feel like another diet plan, and I would ultimately get off it and overeat. It was like I couldn't control myself. It was like a light switch would turn on, and I would be off any diet or eating plan I was following and begin overeating and gaining weight. It never occurred to me to connect what was happening in my life (or in my head) at the time to weight gaining. I would reason with myself that the next day I would be back on track, would rationalize that a day or two off the diet was not the end of the world, and all was not lost. The problem with that thinking is that once I was off my diet, I was off for months. The whole time feeling ashamed and guilty and feeling like a loser. How can I not lose weight and keep it off? I had so many nutrition degrees!!!!

> ### *Knowing how to eat healthy does not necessarily mean you will do it.*

Diets bring on more weight. The only thing you end up losing long term is your self-esteem. The cycle of deprivation, and then overeating, makes you regain your weight and perhaps gain more weight than you had lost. Does this sound familiar? Look back on your life and answer the following questions:

1. How many diets have you tried?

2. How much weight have you lost and then regained?

3. How much money and energy have you wasted on one quick fix after another?

4. What was the result? Did any one of them help you get to your goal and stay there? Don't even answer that. You wouldn't be reading this book if your answer was *yes*.

However, come this Monday, or the Monday after that, you will embark on another diet. The diet that promises you to be the answer to your weight struggles. The diet, which if you follow exactly (and you will this time, you really will!), will get you into your pants that haven't fit you in 5 years, or will get you to wear a bikini on your next vacation. Why do women, all over the world, continue to try one diet after another, without success, hoping that the next one will be the last? Would you bake a cake that was inedible, over and over, using the same techniques and ingredients, hoping that this time it would magically taste good? Is there anything else in your life you do that has failed over and over again, yet you continue to do it the exact same way? The answer is likely, "No." You are using the wrong solution to solve your problem! And who do you blame? Yourself! You blame yourself for being weak, when in fact you are just using the wrong methods. You are not broken. You are just stuck in the yo-yo cycle of dieting.

Weight loss marketers are banking on the fact that you will fail at your diet. How else will they make money on the "next best thing?"

So, what about a healthy eating plan, you say? A plan that will balance my meals, not deprive me of my nutritional requirements—what about that? This is what most Registered Dietitians will do for you. Dietitians know a lot about food and nutrition. In fact, we are the experts in the field. If you want to know the latest research in the field of nutrition, ask a Dietitian. To become a Dietitian, you have to obtain a 4-year University Degree in Science or Applied Science, followed by a 1 year internship or a Master's Degree. We are also held to very high standards and have to be in good standing with our College, as well as continuously improving our skills through continuing education. Dietitians don't only see clients who need to lose weight. Dietitians also counsel people of all ages with a myriad of conditions. However, when it comes to helping people who have been on one diet or another, tried one eating plan after another, with no long-term success, Dietitians are not using the right recipe. We just weren't taught this in school. Dietitians want to help and they are doing everything they can and know so they can help you succeed. But it's like baking a cake and leaving out the flour and the eggs, and only adding milk, sugar, and baking soda. Good luck! Until I realized that achieving the weight you want has very little to do with only focusing on the food you eat, and until I came up with my system that WILL work, I didn't know any better. I just knew that my clients were not keeping their weight off long term and were beating themselves up with each failure. I also knew that I was losing and regaining the same 10–15 pounds, over and over and over.

> ***Achieving your best weight has little to do with focusing on every morsel of food that goes into your mouth.***

No Such Thing as Willpower

Willpower. **That** word. That judgmental word that determines if you've been naughty or good. That word that you are constantly using to gage how you are feeling. When a colleague brought donuts to work, did you exercise willpower and not eat one? Yes? Good... No? You have no willpower. What does the word *willpower* mean to you? How does this word define who you think you are as a person, and how does it define what kind of day you are having? Does willpower mean you are strong? Competent? Successful? Worthy of being loved? Does having *lack* of willpower mean you are useless? Weak? A failure? Undeserving? Let's think about this for a moment. Are you allowing a single word to determine whether you are a good person or not?

Allowing a word to determine whether you speak nicely to yourself or not? Allowing to base your self-worth on one word? This may shock you, but there is no such thing as willpower. There is no "WILLpower" and there is no "WON'Tpower." Willpower is really just conscious or mental focus to resist temptation, and you have to be continuously and intently focused on that something to keep seeing results. This determined focus will work as long as you can hold it. Keep in mind that when you are focused on anything so intently, the rest of your life gets much less attention. That will work in the short term, until everything else you've been neglecting comes to bite you in the butt.

There is no such thing as willpower.

This is so true in dieting. When you start your new diet, you are extremely motivated and you give it your full attention. You are so motivated that it is easy for you to say *no* to tempting foods, the foods that just yesterday you were eating right out of the bag. In the beginning, it requires minimal effort to follow a diet plan, no matter how restrictive. You are at peak motivation, following your diet and beginning to see some results. However, as time goes on, that constant negative chatter in your head, which you may be completely unaware of (but more on that later), is making it increasingly difficult to avoid using food as your crutch to feel better. You also realize that you have been neglecting other areas of your life that require your attention (like your children, your husband, your friends, even the laundry), so your dieting focus begins to dwindle. You are actually fighting with yourself, without necessarily knowing it. You are fighting against your inner beliefs and habits. Your motivation begins to diminish and it requires more and more effort to stay motivated. It is very difficult and exhausting to be constantly struggling with yourself and to exude such willpower for a long time toward anything.

> ## *Your inner struggle is exhausting.*

As your focus and motivation decreases, so does your success. Other aspects of your life, which are equally important to you, compete with the energy you have been spending on following your diet. This is the time where you "lose" your willpower or give in to temptation, so your motivation and focus continue to drop, and your progress slows down until it completely stalls. Once your progress stalls, the motivation is gone. Once the motivation is gone, the focus goes as well. What's left? No motivation and no focus sends you right back to your old habits. The overeating, the bingeing, the continuously filling yourself up with food. This continues until you are again at that place. That place where nothing fits and you are disgusted with yourself. That place where you can't take it another day. This is usually the time you start to recall how motivated you were when you went on your last diet. If only you could go back to that place again. If only you could again be so motivated and focused—that would solve all of your weight issues! So what do you do? You start another diet. This is your yo-yo dieting cycle. This mindful awareness is the first step in breaking this cycle and help you stop blaming and judging yourself so harshly.

One Brain, Two Minds

Why is it that you are so motivated when you start a new diet but lose motivation as time goes on? It's actually very simple: your mind gets in the way. As do your old habits.

Do you ever wonder why you end up doing the exact opposite of what you set out to do? Do you ever wonder why you end up eating half a box of cookies after you told yourself you will only have one? Ever wonder how you can do things so opposite of what you promised yourself you would do? Do you ever get the feeling you are just doing things on automatic pilot, as if you don't have any control? Well, the good news is that you are not going crazy and you do not have a personality disorder. You are completely normal. It is just your Unconscious Mind doing its job.

Your mind is composed of two very distinct parts: the Conscious Mind and the Unconscious Mind. Both of these parts serve a purpose.

The Conscious Mind is only 10% of your whole mind and is your present focus and awareness. You use this part of your mind when you are reading a book, doing a math equation, or listening to your friend on the phone. It is the part of your mind that you utilize to make decisions in the present and the part that you use to focus on a task.

Your Unconscious Mind is the other 90% of your mind. Your Unconscious Mind controls all of your bodily functions like breathing and blinking, your heart beating, and digestion of your food. Can you imagine the chaos if you had to remember to take a breath, expand your lungs, or make your heart beat? You'd never get anything done! Your Unconscious Mind is also your memory bank. You can think of your Unconscious Mind as a large filing cabinet filled with many folders, each one with many sheets of paper. All of your past experiences and memories are stored there. This is where you keep all of your habits, values, and emotions, as well as what you believe about the world and what you believe to be true about yourself. Both positive and negative emotions and experiences are kept there. The Unconscious Mind likes to keep things status quo. Any big change in your normal patterns and actions is considered a threat. The ultimate goal of the Unconscious Mind is to protect you; however, it can also keep you stuck in an old habit or belief that is not serving you well and is keeping you from achieving your goals, no matter how much you think you want them.

> ## *Your Unconscious Mind wants to keep things the way they are.*

Before the age of 7, information flows between the two parts of the mind quite easily without filtering. Children readily believe in Santa Claus or the Easter Bunny. Just try telling them they can't be a Super Hero when they grow up. It is also at this time that, whatever we hear from our parents, teachers, caregivers, and any other people who make an impact in our lives, we tend to believe. So, if you were told you were stupid and wouldn't amount to anything in your life, you may end up believing it. This can then become part of your limiting beliefs. After age 7, once you start maturing and can look at life more critically, the filter between the two minds gets thicker. This filter is called the Critical Faculty. Imagine this being like a Doorman at an expensive hotel who decides who to let in and who to keep out. You can visualize your Conscious Mind outside the hotel, and your Unconscious Mind is inside the hotel, behind the Doorman. The job of the Doorman is to keep people who do not belong in the hotel out of the hotel. The same happens with your mind and what gets to your Unconscious Mind. Anything that does not match its beliefs (even negative beliefs that are keeping you stuck) is kept out and not allowed in.

> ## *The Critical Faculty is like a Doorman, keeping information out that it perceives does not belong.*

This can be useful and harmful at the same time. If I tell you to jump off an airplane so you can fly like a bird, this will not match your unconscious programming that you have. You know that you cannot fly and will likely die if you follow through with my request. This is useful! The Doorman is doing a good job. The Doorman can also, however, keep you stuck in a habit or belief that is no longer working for you—a belief you no longer want, a habit you wish to break.

Elizabeth J.

Take Elizabeth J., for example. Elizabeth came to me to help her lose weight. She was looking for the perfect diet to lose the extra weight once and for all. She had tried at least 10 different diets in her life and all resulted in the same outcome: she would lose 10–25 pounds (depending on how long she could follow it), and would inevitably become bored with the diet and return to her old eating habits. This always resulted in her putting the weight back on. Elizabeth felt that she just hadn't found that perfect diet. Elizabeth came to me highly motivated to start a new diet plan, as she was going away in 1 month to Mexico and wanted to fit into her bathing suit.

During our detailed assessment session, Elizabeth revealed that she always finished all the food on her plate. She would even finish the food off of her kids' plates after they were done with their meals. It didn't matter if she was hungry or full; she automatically ate the rest of the food off the plates as she was cleaning up after dinner.

When Elizabeth was young, meal times were a battle. She had a lot of pressure put upon her by her parents to finish every morsel of food that was placed in front of her. Her parents would make her stay at the table until her plate was completely clean. She sometimes sat for hours at the kitchen table playing with the food, not wanting to eat it. Elizabeth was not allowed to leave the table until she ate the food. You might say that her parents were abusive, and you may have experienced a similar type of parenting when you were growing up. Her parents were parenting her the best way they knew how. They grew up during the war when food was scarce and it was a sin to throw food away. They wanted their daughter, Elizabeth, to grow up healthy and well nourished. When Elizabeth would finally eat the food left for her, she would be greatly praised about how wonderful it was that she had finished her food, and how happy she had made her parents. Elizabeth's Unconscious Mind was taking this all in. The connection between cleaning off the plate and being good and loved, was made in her mind. It happened over and over and over. The more an event is repeated and the stronger the emotion that accompanies that event, the more it will result in the connection being made.

So now, Elizabeth is all grown up with a family of her own, struggles to lose weight, continues to finish everything on her plate, and her kids' plates. She is doing this because unconsciously this is how she feels she is good enough. This is how she feels loved. Elizabeth does this automatically. There is no thought involved. She is meeting the need of feeling good and loved the only way she knows how—by eating.

When Elizabeth starts a new diet, she only uses the 10% of her mind (the Conscious Mind) to exert great focus and determination. That's where she is feeling she has willpower and motivation. However, her need to feel loved (which she feels when she eats, and overeats, without listening to her hunger cues) will be a much stronger force than the 10% of her mind. This need will override any attempt or focus, because it will be coming from her Unconscious Mind—the 90%.

Can you see why all of Elizabeth's previous diets failed? Putting Elizabeth on a diet plan or a healthy eating plan will only work short term. Food provides her with a feeling of being loved.

The more an event is repeated, the higher the chance that a connection will be made in your brain.

During our coaching sessions, we explored other ways that Elizabeth can feel good about herself and feel loved. Ways that have nothing to do with food. We also eliminated her limiting belief that she requires food to feel loved. Once the Unconscious Mind can get its needs met in other ways (feeling loved and feeling that she is good enough), ways which are healthier for Elizabeth, the issue of why she is overeating and using food improperly disappears!

Now that you have learned that there is no such thing as willpower and that your Unconscious Mind holds the answers of why you are still struggling with dieting, it's time to learn how to shift your focus to getting what you actually want.

Chapter 2

Where Is Your Focus?

What You See Is All In Your Head

We are bombarded by over 2 million bits of information per second which enter our nervous system through the five senses that make up our sensory input channels. These senses include Visual (what we see); Auditory (what we hear); Kinesthetic (what we feel); Olfactory (what we smell); and Gustatory (what we taste)[1]. Just think about all the details in your life as you go on about your day. From the pebbles on the ground, to the leaves on the trees, to the colour differences of every brick of the houses you pass. The amount of stimuli is overwhelming! Most of this information that is presented to us gets filtered in our mind. If we didn't filter it in some way, we'd go bonkers. Imagine being given 2 million apples that you had to look at and identify, but you only had one second to do it, because 2 million more would come at you the next second. That is a lot of data and stimuli coming to you at one time, and we can't take all of it in. We end up processing only about 134 bits of information per second. That is a lot less than what is available! That is much less than 1%!

To help us deal with all of this incoming data, we delete, distort, and generalize it. *Deleting* means that we don't even see some of this information, as if it wasn't there. Deleting allows you to focus on what

---

[1] *The NLP Communication Model, developed by Tad James & Wyatt Woodsmall (1988) from the work of Richard Bandler & John Grinder (1975).*

is important to you at the time and ignore what is not. When you are preparing dinner, you can focus on the meal preparation and can ignore the birds chirping outside or the number of tiles on the floor. This is good, because it allows you to complete your tasks. The problem lies when we delete what is actually important to us and what we should have paid attention to. For example, if you think that the teenagers living across the street are trouble makers, you will only notice their actions that are in agreement with that statement. You will notice that they are rowdy late at night or play their music too loudly. You will not notice anything that contradicts your belief. You will not see them helping their Mom carry groceries into the house or walking with their elderly grandparent.

Distorting means changing the information so that it fits in to what you believe to be true. Distorting is useful unless you do it only to be right. If you colour your hair and your kids still recognize you, they are distorting their reality of their image of you and will still realize that it is you. This is good, or else you would have a lot of convincing to do to make sure they know you are their Mom. On the downside, distorting can have a negative impact on how you feel. Have you ever left a voicemail for someone and were waiting for a call back, and the person did not respond for a few days? You then started inventing all of the reasons why the person was not calling you back, such as them being mad at you, or that they don't think you are important enough for them to call you. In the end, when they did call you, it turned out they were on vacation and didn't hear the voicemail until they returned. The problem with distorting information is that we distort it to fit into how we feel, what we say to ourselves, and how we believe the world functions. Another way to say it is that we make it fit into our perception of the world.

Generalizing can also be helpful to us or be a hinder to us. For example, we know that a spoon is a tool we use to help us eat. So, any spoon—silver, gold, pewter, with a wide handle or a slim handle—is still a spoon. We have generalized all spoons into this category and whenever we come across a spoon, we know what it is used for. This saves us a lot of time relearning every single element that we come in contact with. On the downside, generalizing can keep us stuck in the same spot. Imagine you were stung by a bee when you were a child. Now, every time you see a bee, you think that you will be stung. You now have a phobia, even though the event only happened one time. You have generalized that every time you come into contact with a bee, you will be stung. Or maybe, when you were in school, you had to present in front of the class; you were nervous, forgot what to say about your topic, felt embarrassed, and ended up getting a lower grade. You may generalize to say that you are a bad presenter and cannot speak in front of a group.

We delete, distort, or generalize information that comes to us based on filters such as language, values, beliefs, memories, attitudes, and decisions. These filters are deep in our programming and something we don't consciously think about, but they rule our lives. Values and beliefs are very important and determine what we base our lives on and how we conduct ourselves. For example, trust may be a very important value to you, and so the life decisions you make, the friends you have, and the type of life you want to lead will be based on this value. Any information that comes through these filters, we form a picture or a movie in our heads (based on pictures, feelings, sounds, smells, tastes and self-talk). Let me ask you what you think of Brussels Sprouts— do you love them or do you hate them? How did you represent them to yourself? Was it in picture form or did you have a taste of them in your mouth? Did you say to yourself, "Gross," or "Yummy?" However, you reacted to the question, you made an internal image in your head. Once you formed a picture, your actual physiology may have changed. You may have contorted your face if you hate Brussels Sprouts or started salivating if you love them. This will then have an impact on your behaviour—what you say and do— as well as your future experience. So, whatever has an impact on your mind, will affect the body as well. Whatever has an impact on the body, will affect the mind.

How would you feel if you could alter your filters to achieve all that you want to achieve? To have an effect on any of your unwanted or unhealthy behaviours which prevent you from living the life that you want? Well, you can. In fact, you already have the ability and all of the resources you need to succeed. All you are missing is the vessel—the vessel to take you from your current island of unsatisfaction and despair to the island of magnificence and success.

The More You Focus On Your Weight, The More Weight You Gain

Does the title above seem opposite of what should happen? Doesn't focus produce change? Remember what you read in Chapter 1 about focus and willpower? The determined focus while you are using your Conscious Mind (the 10% of your total mind) will only yield results while you focus on it and ignore everything else. This is something you can't sustain for a long period of time. In addition, what you focus on, you get more of. When you think about the extra weight that you are carrying around, you are focused on that extra weight. Thus you get more of it! When you are incessantly thinking about your pants being tight and uncomfortable, guess what? Your pants will continue to feel snug and uncomfortable! Obsessing about the numbers on the scale being too high? You will continue to see those numbers. In fact, they may even continue to increase.

Let's look at another example to explain this that is not related to weight. Ever notice how some people with money troubles continue to have bad luck and money troubles, and other people appear to receive money from every angle? They get promotions at work, win prizes in raffles, and make fruitful decisions in the stock market? Everything they touch turns to gold. You may say that they are "lucky." How can one person be so lucky and another person so unlucky? People who are in debt, put all of their energy and effort into thinking about that debt. And the result? They get more of it. The pipes in their house freeze during the winter and burst; every month there is a new expense not accounted for; and the debt continues to increase. What about those "lucky" people? They assume that they will continue to attract money and good things will come their way. They put their energy and thought into positivity, so that is what they get. The "unlucky" people are so determined to only think of their negative situation, that even if a positive situation was staring them in the face, they would miss it. Those "unlucky" people would not even hear the announcement about a job promotion coming up.

The same situation happens with weight loss. You are putting all of your energy into what you do *not* want. You are so focused on your excess weight, your inability to exercise self-control, and your bingeing, that you get more of it. More of what you don't want. Ever hear the saying, "What you focus on expands?" (No pun intended.) You end up putting out into the world that you want more weight.

When you put all of your energy and time and money into what you do not want (your extra weight), you are only focusing on your problem. You are not even facing the solution. Your "problem" (the extra weight) is in front of you, staring you so close in the face, and your back is completely turned away from the solution. That is why you don't see it. It's behind you. You can't help but be unsuccessful when the solution is so far and behind you. You need to turn yourself around and look at the solution, and turn your back to the problem. If you begin to put your time and energy, and money, into your solution, that is what you will get more of in your life.

Have you ever heard the notion that everything you want in life, everything you can imagine, is right in front of you and you just have to grab it? The problem is that if you are not seeing it, or hearing it, you will ignore it. Any opportunity that will lead you to success will be ignored by you, as if it's not even there. Remember all of the stimuli and information we are bombarded with every second of every day? It's so much more than we can handle, and we end up with a much smaller chunk of information that we are able to process. Well, if you are so intent on focusing on the extra pounds that you are carrying and how much you hate yourself for it, you will pick out evidence from your daily life that is in line with your thinking. By focusing on what you don't want, your mind then filters and absorbs this negative stimuli and information. As a result, you get more of it. Throughout your day, you will find ways to reinforce the fact that you are a failure and that you have no self-control. This will lead you to overeat, and you get to prove that you were right.

> **Whatever you focus on expands, so focus on the solution, not the problem.**

The Reticular Activating System –
Your Personal Private Detective

How awesome would it be if your mind could pick out and notice all the incoming data in your life that you require to be successful? Would you like to have your very own Private Detective who does the job for you and guides your attention to help you achieve your goals? Once you have specific goals in mind (we will discuss goal setting later in this book), you will actually be helping your mind to pay close attention to your surroundings and hand pick information that will help you accomplish your goals.

This can be achieved with the help of The Reticular Activating System (RAS). RAS is a bundle of nerves sitting densely in the back of the central core in the brain stem and is responsible for different functions in the body. One of its functions is to filter out information (images, sounds, etc.) that we are constantly bombarded with, day in and day out, and bring relevant information to your attention. It will bring into your conscious mind only the information that is of interest to you. Remember that you are only processing 134 bits of information per second (with your Conscious Mind), whereas there are over 2million bits of information coming at you (and your Unconscious Mind) at any given second.

Here is a simple example to illustrate this. Have you ever bought a car and, after driving off the lot, you begin to see that exact same model of car on the road repeatedly, as if a lot of people decided to purchase the same type of car, and it is now the most popular car to drive? Is this actually the case? Of course not; but because you have bought this car and it is something that is of focus and interest to you, your brain let's this particular information into your Conscious Mind and you become aware of it. A month before you bought your car, you didn't notice all the similar cars on the road, and now you do. Nothing in your physical environment has changed. How you process information and what you focus on, has. Everything you need to be successful is there for your taking. You just haven't established it yet. Once you do, your senses (eyes, ears, brain) will help you find it.

When you are specific about what it is you want, and you visualize it frequently, you are sending a message to your Conscious Mind and Unconscious Mind what is of interest and significance to you. By programming the RAS on what in your environment to focus on, out of all the data you are bombarded with, you will achieve your goal. By setting goals, which we will discuss later, you can program your RAS to purposely focus on what you want so that you will notice the resources, people, and opportunities that you need. What is YOUR solution? What is your goal? We will discuss goal setting in Chapter 7 but, for now, let me just say that anything you put your energy toward has to be positive, and stated as something you DO want, not something you DON'T want.

The RAS can also help you NOT achieve your goals. If you continuously say to yourself that you are a failure and will never be "slim" or "healthy," or that exercising is too hard, the RAS will help you to see that this is true by bringing focus to factors in your life that will reinforce your thoughts, and your Unconscious Mind will make sure that you achieve your goal of being "a failure."

You now know that by focusing on your solution, you can activate your Private Detective to assist you in bringing to your attention information that will get you to your success; it is time to uncover your deep-rooted, limiting beliefs that have been keeping you stuck.

Chapter 3

Getting To The Bottom Of It All

What's Your Excuse?

Sometimes we blame external situations or other people for the predicament we are in. Ask yourself the question of why you are overweight, or why every diet you have been on has failed? How many excuses can you come up with? How many people can you blame? Is it because you don't have time to exercise? Is it because your kids won't eat vegetables, so you don't prepare them? Is it because you are mad at your husband, so you eat two bowls of ice-cream? Are you blaming your parents who only gave you dessert after you finished your whole meal and have taught you to not listen to your hunger and satiety signals? Is your boss stressing you out?

Now, I'm not saying you haven't been dealt a difficult deck of cards in your life, whether in childhood or in adulthood. I don't know anyone who has not experienced difficulty in their lives. Nevertheless, are you still blaming someone for the life that you lead now? Are you still living in your past and trying to change your past so that you can change your present?

Who are you blaming for your weight?

Are you the Driver in your life or the Passenger? Let's take a look at characteristics of both.

The Passenger in a car has little control over the roads that are chosen on the trip, the speed of the vehicle, or the turns and exits taken. The only thing the Passenger can do is whine and complain to the driver that he is going too fast or too slow, or taking the long way to get to the destination. The Passenger has completely relinquished his control in this situation.

Now let's look at the Driver. The Driver decides on the speed driven and which route to take. If the Driver sees that there is construction up ahead and all the cars are at a standstill, he can decide to take another route.

Situations in our lives, both positive and negative, happen all the time. How you react to these situations, and the meaning you give them, is in your complete control. What?!?! You might think: "How can I be responsible for my boss providing a stressful job environment? How can I be responsible for my kids pushing my buttons? How can I prevent my husband from bringing home cookies when he knows I can't say no? How can I not get mad if my mother-in-law comes over unannounced?" Who are you blaming for how you feel and your behaviour? You are right; you may not be able to prevent some of these situations. But you know what you can have complete control over? How you react to these situations. That is in your complete control. So, if your boss makes your job environment stressful and you decide to deal with it by eating a bag of chips, that is on you. What are you using food for? No amount of food will satisfy your emotional needs.

As long as you continue to use excuses and blame others for why you are not living the life you want, you will continue to be stuck where you are now. Only by becoming the Driver in your life, will you be able to have lasting change.

For the next week, write down different situations that happen in your life, how you behaved, and what the result was. Did you behave as the Driver or the Passenger? Record even the smallest events that may seem completely unimportant. If you arrived late to work on Monday morning, who did you blame? Did you blame the slow car in front of you? Hitting every red light? Or maybe you realized that you need to start getting out of bed 20 minutes earlier instead of pressing the snooze button.

Keep a list of every event for one week and see if there is a pattern. What triggers you to become a Passenger in your life? What makes you behave like the victim in a situation, feeling like you have no control? Think of what you can do next time to get the control back into your life. Remember you may not be able to change everything that happens to you, but you can always change how you see the situation and react to the situation. This exercise should give you great awareness of how you respond to unpleasant situations and what you can do to become the Driver in your life. Once you realize that you CAN be the Driver in your life, and of your life, you will become more empowered, and begin to behave differently, continuously altering your course of action and reaching any goals you set out for yourself.

> **The Driver has control over every situation.**

Jackie E.

Jackie E. came to see me to help her lose 30 pounds. She had tried numerous diets in her life but could not stick to a diet plan for more than 3 weeks. She was unhappy and frustrated and was tired of missing out on life. During our assessment, it quickly became clear that Jackie saw herself as the Passenger in many situations in her life. As a Real Estate agent, a lot of her working hours were spent on the road. She daily stopped at fast food restaurants to grab a high calorie, greasy lunch. At times, she would come home late in the evening and be too tired to start cooking, so she would pop something frozen into the microwave, grab a can of pop, and then have a large bowl of ice-cream for dessert. Late evening was a time when Jackie could finally unwind and catch up on her favourite shows, which she liked to do while eating her dinner and snacking. Her last dieting attempt included skipping breakfast, followed by an apple for a snack and a salad with a small piece of chicken breast at dinner. She had no idea of what she could eat for lunch if it didn't include fast food. After a week, Jackie felt so lethargic and tired and hungry that she went right back to overeating. She blamed her crazy working hours for keeping her from having a routine she could follow.

Many questions during my assessment with Jackie would be followed by: "I can't do that because..." Responding with, "I can't because...," is a great way to keep you stuck exactly where you are. It means that you are not the Driver in your life, and you are not ready to put your full effort into getting to your goal.

During the first visit with Jackie, I knew she wouldn't be successful at reaching her goal because she did not see herself as the Driver. Her excuses would continue to be a barrier to her success. She was not ready to take full responsibility for her life. Remember, difficult situations will arise. How you deal with them, and what you do about them, is what's important and what makes you the Driver of your life. After I explained this to Jackie, she was adamant that she needed my help. I sent Jackie home with a lot of tasks and plans of action to see if she would be able to move from being the Passenger to being the Driver. Two weeks later, we met again; I am happy to report she was able to now realize that her excuses were keeping her from attaining her goals. She stopped blaming her job and time schedule for being the reason why she couldn't do something. We were then able to continue with our coaching sessions because I knew she would be successful.

Readiness Checklist

Read the following statements in the list below to assess your readiness to take control over your life!

1. If you are willing to stop waiting for the "perfect diet" and do something different, you are ready!

2. If you are willing to do the techniques outlined in this book, you are ready!

3. If you are willing to take responsibility for your actions and anything that happens to you, you are ready!

4. If you are willing to set goals and take action, you are ready!

5. If you are willing to be uncomfortable for a short time, in order to gain great successes and rewards, you are ready!

If I Just Ate, Why Am I Still Hungry?

Think about your last few meals or snacks—did you pay attention to what you were eating, or were you eating without having any awareness of the food or to whether you were hungry or not? How often do you continue eating when you are already full? How often do you look at the bag of chips you were consuming and are surprised to find the bag almost empty? What kinds of things are you saying to yourself when you eat? What kinds of sensations is your body feeling? Anxiety? Nervousness? Is there something in your life that you are expecting food to satisfy? Before we go further into this, I'd like you to answer the following questions:

1. What's Your Crutch?

When it comes to your weight and dieting, what is it that is keeping you from living the life you want? Using the space below, write out in a sentence or two what problem you would like to be rid of. Remember that you need to be the Driver of your life in stating the problem. If you think that the problem of your weight is the fact that your mother-in-law makes killer, deep fried donuts and brings them to your house, and that is the problem, you are in Passenger mode. Make the statement about you. Is your crutch similar to the one I had, that you are constantly either dieting or gaining weight (yo-yo dieting)? Are you bingeing at night after the kids have gone to bed? Are you driving from one fast food joint to another throughout the day? Are you a sneaky eater and hide your overeating by eating in the car, or at other times when you are alone?

An example may be: "I eat junk food in the evening until my stomach hurts so much I can barely move." Whatever it may be, write it down in the space below.

_____
_____
_____
_____

2. Go back to the beginning

When you think back to how long you have been struggling with weight issues and dieting, how far back can you remember? Was it before puberty? As a teenager? In your 20s, or later? Think of the first time you decided your body was not good enough and you had to lose weight.

_____
_____
_____

3. Holding you back

When you think about your answer in #1, has that problem been holding you back from doing or experiencing anything in your life? Do you find you often say things to yourself like, "when I lose the weight, I will _____" (insert action). For example: "When I lose 20 pounds, I will put a profile on a dating site; When I lose 30 pounds, I will start being more social and go out more often; When I fit into my skinny jeans, I will leave the job I have now, which I hate, and start to look for my dream job; When I like how I look, I will finally be able to have a better relationship with my husband." Is there anything you are not doing now because you are not at your goal weight? Write the answer below.

_____

_____

_____

_____

Here is something I would like you to consider. It is highly possible that whatever your extra weight is holding you back from doing is the exact reason you continue to sabotage yourself and remain overweight! In my case, having a private coaching practice was something I always wanted to have, but I decided that until I got a handle on my own eating issues, it was not something I could embark on. Unconsciously, I was also afraid that I would not be successful at running my own business. So, I sabotaged all efforts at overcoming my eating struggles, which would keep me stuck in my distorted eating, and then I would never have to face the possibility of failing. I spent all my time so "busy" focusing on my weight and dieting, and thinking that it was my biggest issue in life, that I didn't have the time or energy to take action on what it would take to run a successful coaching business. As long as I was not doing anything toward my business, I had no chance of failing and proving myself right—being "not good enough" was my unconscious self-limiting belief.

> *Using all of your focus and energy worrying about your weight keeps you busy so that you don't have to take action toward something you really want, and face possible failure.*

Sally J.

Sally J. was a 27-year old single girl who came to see me to help her lose 45 pounds. Sally had not had a romantic relationship for a few years and wanted to start dating again. She determined she would need to put a profile on an online dating site as a way to meet any prospects. She wanted to first to lose the extra weight before embarking on finding her Prince Charming. Sally was a "sneaky eater." She ate average sized and even smaller than regular portions of foods when in front of people; however, once she was alone, she would overeat on snack foods like chips and cookies. This would inevitably lead to Sally feeling disgusted with herself and she would start dieting. Sally had been a chronic dieter since she was a teen-ager and whatever weight she lost, always came back.

During our sessions, I uncovered that Sally's unconscious, self-limiting belief was that she thought she was "unlovable."

Sally J. grew up in a family with 3 sisters and 1 brother. She felt that her brother, being the only boy, was given preferential treatment by her parents (at least in her young eyes at the time). Her brother was allowed to do many things Sally and her sisters were not; he was allowed to climb trees in the backyard, run outside with his friends at a young age without supervision, and seemed to receive more attention from their parents. It's possible that Sally's parents were just more overprotective over their daughters because they were girls, and her brother received more attention because he was often getting himself into trouble and did not listen to their parents well, whereas Sally and her sisters were more quiet and obedient. In Sally's young mind, she concluded that her brother was loved more than she was and that there must be something wrong with her; she must be unlovable.

> ***You may be unconsciously sabotaging your efforts so you don't have to face the limiting belief you hold about yourself.***

The adult Sally consciously wanted to have that significant other in her life; however, unconsciously, she didn't feel that she deserved it. In her mind, being loveable meant looking a certain way, which was slim. Furthermore, if she lost the weight and then met someone she liked, she may have to face the fact that he would not reciprocate her feelings, thus reinforcing her belief of being unlovable. As long as Sally remained overweight and focused on her struggles with that, she wouldn't have to face the possibility that her biggest unconscious belief and fear (being unlovable) was true.

Uncover Your Unconscious Self-Limiting Belief

As you can see from the previous section, you do not have to have gone through a traumatic experience in your childhood to have an unconscious self-limiting belief. All that was required was to have absorbed information around you from a child's perspective—whether from your parents, your teachers, caregivers, or even television—and then to have made a decision about yourself. The more that information or event was repeated (in Sally's case, her parents paying more attention to her brother), specifically when it evoked emotion in you, the stronger the belief became. It was then sealed in your

Unconscious Mind and, now as an adult, only the information that is aligned to your unconscious self-limiting beliefs will by-pass the Critical Faculty (the Doorman) into your Unconscious Mind. Everything else, no matter how much you may want it consciously, will just bounce right off, like a rubber ball.

Do the following exercise to help uncover your unconscious self-limiting belief:

1. In the space below, write down the exact goal you want to achieve when it comes to your weight. For example, "I want to fit into my size 4 jeans;" or "I want to weigh 140 pounds."

_____

_____

_____

_____

2. Now think about all of the reasons and barriers keeping you from reaching your goal. The reasons have to be about you and to do with you. Start the sentences with "I" statements. So, if your goal is to lose 50 pounds, you could write: "I can't lose 50 pounds because....."

List as many reasons as you can think of. Once you have your initial list, ask yourself the question again and see if you come up with more reasons. Stop when you can't come up with any new reasons.

The first few reasons you come up with will be more at your conscious level, such as "I don't know what I'm supposed to eat," or "I don't have time to cook healthy foods." They are at your conscious level because you are able to verbalize them rather quickly. Keep asking the question of how that is a problem for you. I don't want you to judge your answers, I just want you to keep answering the question, "How is that a problem for me?" until you to get at those self-limiting beliefs which come from your Unconscious Mind and are sabotaging your efforts of success. Write all the reasons below.

_____
_____
_____
_____
_____
_____
_____
_____
_____
_____
_____
_____
_____
_____
_____
_____

You know you have uncovered your unconscious self-limiting beliefs when you get to one or more of the three answers:

1. **I am unlovable** (I can't be loved; Nobody will want me; I will be alone)

2. **I am not good enough/I am not worthy** (I am a loser; I can't do anything right; I'm a failure)

3. **I am powerless** (I have no voice; I can't speak my mind; I am weak)

Everyone in this world, no matter what their background, socioeconomic status, education level, or where they were born, will have at least one of these self-limiting beliefs. A decision about these unconscious self-limiting beliefs was made as a young child, through a young child's experience and perception of the workings of the world.

> **You adopted your unconscious self-limiting beliefs when you made a decision about yourself as a young child.**

Let me illustrate what happened during an assessment with Liza K., a 45- year old woman who had been struggling with dieting for 20 years:

Me: Liza, please tell me why you are here.

Liza: I don't know what to eat anymore. I don't know which diet I should try next. Nothing seems to work.

Me: Anything else?

Liza: I have been on so many diets, and I just can't seem to stick to any one for longer than 1 month. I end up regaining all the weight that I lose and even more.

Me: Anything else?

Liza: No, that's all.

Me: Can you please tell me why it's an issue for you that you can't stick to a diet and you end up regaining the weight?

Liza: Because I hate how I look. My clothes are tight on me. I hate buying new clothes and I dread going on vacation because I have to wear a bathing suit.

Me: And why is that an issue for you that your clothes are tight and you hate how you look?

Liza: If my clothes don't fit me, it means I am fat.

Me: How is that an issue for you to be fat?

Liza: I don't want my husband to look at me. I never let him see me undressed.

Me: And how is that an issue?

Liza: He gets upset that I don't want him to be near me and this negatively impacts our relationship.

Me: And how is having a poor relationship with your husband a problem for you?

Liza: If our relationship is bad, he will look for someone else to be with.

Me: And if he looks for someone else, how is that an issue for you?

Liza: It means he doesn't love me, I don't deserve to be loved, he will leave me, and then I will be all alone.

Me: Thank you Liza.

Liza's unconscious self-limiting belief was that she was unlovable.

Now that you have learned why it's important to be the Driver in your life and have uncovered the deep limiting beliefs about yourself that are keeping you from moving forward, it is time to focus on your negative self-talk, your thoughts and your feelings.

Chapter 4

Moving Toward Success

The Mean Girl

We often eat on automatic and berate ourselves for eating after the fact. Sometimes the cravings and the urge to eat are so strong, it is as if we have been taken over by a madman. I cannot tell you the number of times I would go to the grocery store, buy a few pastries, and rip into the bag as soon as I got into the car. I would then finish all of them in a matter of minutes, and get rid of the evidence before I got home.

If you pay very close attention, just before you grab that bag of chips or pastries, there are a bunch of thoughts or pictures or voices going through your head that are then followed by the action of grabbing that food. What are they? Did anything happen earlier in the day to make you want to grab those chips? Think back to a recent time when you mindlessly ate something even though you were not hungry—a time where you felt you were out of control with your eating. What were you thinking just before that? Were you saying anything to yourself? Did you see any pictures? Did you hear anybody else's voice saying something to you?

For me, when I started to pay close attention to what my negative self-talk was, I heard the following:

"You should have been slim by now."

"If you wouldn't have regained the weight, you would have been skinny."

"You can't do anything right."

"You are a farce with all of your nutrition degrees."

I call these voices my *Mean Girl*. These are just some examples of what the Mean Girl inside my head was saying to me. Listening to the Mean Girl only lead me to eat more. Which in turn would make me feel worse. Which would lead me to eat more. It was a vicious cycle that kept me stuck in my problem.

The Mean Girl voice you have inside your head may seem like it's been there forever. In fact, it is likely she's adding her two cents to everything you do, have done, and are thinking of doing. She is scrutinizing your every move, your every thought, your every action. Constantly criticizing you, judging you and putting you down, and using the RAS to filter everything that confirms what she is telling you.

This voice originated from external sources such as parents, teachers, and society in general when you were little. This voice helped keep you safe and in line when you were a child and helped ensure you followed rules: "don't cross the street by yourself; clean your room; don't talk to strangers." As you got older, you would hear this voice whenever you had a thought or took an action. Eventually, you no longer needed your parents to tell you right from wrong because you also had the Mean Girl voice inside you. This is also a time when you adopted your unconscious self-limiting beliefs about yourself (e.g., I'm not good enough; I'm unlovable; I'm not worthy.). Remember how you had no Critical Faculty (Doorman) when you were younger, before age 7? Everything you heard about yourself, and the conclusions you derived, was taken personally into the Unconscious Mind, especially if there was an emotion associated with it. Looking back at your childhood now, you may not understand how you could have come up with the conclusion that you are unlovable, but back then you looked at events from a young child's perspective and life experience.

I'll give you an example from my childhood. My parents (who are wonderful, by the way) continuously reinforced how well I behaved, always listened to them and didn't cause any trouble. They used to call me their "Golden Child." In fact, they would boast about me in front of family members and their friends. Sounds good so far, doesn't it? If I ever behaved in a displeasing manner, I would see the disapproving look in their eyes, and that was enough to let me know I did something wrong. I was a people pleaser and, in my child's mind, I did not ever want to see my parents disappointed. Even back then, I realized I couldn't be perfect and a disappointment at the same time, so I concluded that unless I was perfect, I was not good enough and I was unlovable. As an adult, I can see how faulty that reasoning was. As an adult, I know that having a messy room as a child does not make me less lovable. But that is the connection I made back then. As I grew older, every time I was not perfect (e.g., did not get straight A's; came home past my curfew; didn't clean my room), the Mean Girl inside my head was there to reinforce my negative beliefs. With time, it became a part of my unconscious programming, and the negative voice I heard seemed like it was there forever. I came to own that voice as my own. I hope you see that now that you are an adult, your Mean Girl is not serving you well, is keeping you stuck in your current situation, and is keeping you from reaching your goals and having the life you want and deserve!

What is your Mean Girl telling you? Write down your Mean Girl thoughts below:

_____
_____
_____
_____
_____
_____

Sometimes it is hard to remember our thoughts and feelings after they have passed and we have already finished the cupcakes to make ourselves feel better. If that is the scenario for you, for the next 7 days, I want you to write down everything you are saying to yourself just before you grab that food to satisfy your emotions. Really start to pay attention to the negative voice in your head. The voice of the Mean Girl. This negative self-talk is actually what is keeping you from living your best life (more on that later). Below, write down every time you reach for food for reasons other than hunger, and what you hear or see in your head just before you reach for it.

_____
_____
_____
_____
_____

Confront the Mean Girl

The inner chatter of the Mean Girl keeps you stuck in your yo-yo dieting cycle. The Mean Girl originated from when you were a child and she continues to behave with the maturity and experience of a child. If you recall from what I told you about how you interpret information, you are continuously editing what you see, hear, and feel around you. In fact, you are filtering all information that comes at you so that your Mean Girl seems correct and only reinforces how badly you feel about yourself.

Here are some examples of how your distorted thinking keeps you in alignment with your negative self-talk.

1. You have been following a healthy eating plan and feeling good about yourself all week. You go out to dinner and end up eating dessert. All evening, you are berating yourself how you have no self-control and will never lose weight. The next day your breakfast is a donut and coffee with cream and sugar. This *all or nothing* thinking sets you up for failure every time you feel you are not "perfect." In fact, you completely delete all the times you have been successfully working toward your goal and only focus on the one time you did not. Focusing on your "imperfection" only leads you to overeat, and you get to prove your Mean Girl right.

2. You have been losing 2 pounds every week for the last three weeks. On the fourth week, your scale shows that your weight has not budged and is the same as the week before. You feel like you are failing once again. You continue to focus on the lack of results for this one week, working yourself into a frenzy of uncontrollable eating so you can prove yourself right.

3. "A minute on your lips, forever on your hips" is the mantra you have always believed. It is so unfair that your best friend can eat anything and not put on an ounce. The models you see in magazines and on TV were born with an unfair advantage! You believe that just by looking at pizza, you will gain weight. You send yourself into such a tailspin of unfairness of life that you continuously overeat to prove your theory correct.

4. Your husband brings home ice-cream. Your mother-in-law pops by to bring Eggplant Parmesan. A colleague brings donuts into your office every other day. You feel that if it wasn't for these people sabotaging your efforts, you would be able to lose the weight. You continuously blame people and circumstances around you for why you are not successful.

5. You use words like "always" and "never." For example, "I will *never* lose this weight; I can't go to the gym because something *always* comes up."

These are just a few examples of how your thinking may be distorted based on your self-talk and how you filter what is actually occurring. One way to help align your thinking with reality is to question and confront your Mean Girl.

Go back to the list of the Mean Girl thoughts you have written down and challenge the thoughts with the following questions:

1. Am I seeing the whole picture or only focusing on the negative part so that I can prove my Mean Girl right? Are you only focusing on the fact that you didn't exercise today and forgetting that you have been to the gym 3 times this week? Did you decide that you might as well binge eat because you had 1 cookie and therefore completely sabotaged your healthy eating for that day?

2. How much power does the thought have if I take the emotion out of it? Pretend that it is your best friend who has the Mean Girl thoughts. What would be your advice to her? Taking the emotion out of the thought will give the thought much less power and weight.

3. Am I blaming others for my situation? When I give up my power of being responsible for my life, does it bring me closer to my goal or take me further away from my goal? Remember to be the Driver in your life, not the Passenger.

4. Is this really true? What evidence do I have that this is true? Is it really *always* or *never* true? Have there been instances when this was not true? If you are saying to yourself that you can *never* lose weight, but have actually been able to lose weight in the past, then the word *never* is not true.

5. When I think a situation is unfair, am I only focusing on one part of it? If I look at the whole picture, would I see things differently? Would some people look at my life and see I have an unfair advantage over something that they don't; for example, a wonderful partner, healthy and happy children, a successful career?

6. Do I use the word "should" in my thinking? The word "should" is a judgment word, leaving you feeling disempowered that you did not meet the expectations. What would happen if you change "should" into "could?" For example: "I could go to the gym; I could find the time to cook a healthy meal." Using the word "could" removes the harsh judgment and negative emotion, and provides you with choice.

By continuously paying attention to the Mean Girl's thoughts and confronting the thoughts with the above questions, you will be able to change from a negative emotional state to a positive one.

Whenever your Mean Girl's negative talk comes up, remember that these thoughts stem from child-like beliefs and decisions that were made as a child. It will further help to diminish the power that these thoughts have if you imagine your Mean Girl as a tiny cartoon-like character with a squeaky voice, standing outside your window, speaking in a very muffled tone.

> ***By confronting the Mean Girl,***
> ***you give her less power to dictate your life.***

Think Differently to Feel Differently

Often, my clients believe that how they feel depends solely on what is happening in their external environment. Their husband forgetting to take out the garbage leaves them feeling super annoyed; a friend not returning their phone call makes them angry; a co-worker getting the promotion they wanted brings about feelings of jealousy and not feeling good enough. Ask yourself this question: "Who is *actually* in charge of how I feel?" Let's say you are driving on the highway and another driver cuts you off. How do you react? Do you become angry and blast your horn at them, and then yell at them from your car as you drive by? Do you believe that your anger is a direct result of the other driver's actions and their inability to drive properly?

The fact of the matter is that your anger is not the result of the other driver cutting you off, but it is a direct product of what you were thinking right after the driver cut you off. Your thoughts produced the feeling of anger, which then lead to the action of you honking and screaming at the driver. How you feel at any given moment is directly related to what you are thinking. Why is this important? Because how you behave and, in fact, all of your actions are determined by your feelings, which are a result of your thoughts.

THOUGHTS → FEELINGS → ACTION

How you feel will determine whether you take an action, and it can also keep you *from* taking action. It is very important to understand this concept before you undertake any action. Let's say you made the decision to exercise every morning to help you reach your health and weight loss goals; however, you absolutely hate physical activity. This results in two scenarios: either you get out of bed in the morning when you wake up to your alarm, exercise and hate every minute of it, or you lie in bed making excuses why you can't exercise, until it becomes too late and you have to get ready for work. Until you understand your thoughts and feelings when it comes to being physically active, you will be in a constant struggle with yourself, fighting what you think you should be doing (exercising) with how you feel about exercise (unmotivated, apathetic). Unless you become aware of your thoughts and feelings around physical activity, you will continue to be in conflict with yourself, and will end up giving up.

The same can be said for starting any "diet." Everything we do or don't do depends on our feelings, which are guided by our thoughts. Once you begin to change your thoughts, this will automatically lead to a change in how you feel and, because your feelings determine your actions, you are then able to take action toward what you want in a more effortless and sustainable way.

Let's look at an example of someone who is overweight and is consuming a diet full of unhealthy, greasy, processed foods. They know they should be following a healthier way of eating, that it is better for their overall health, but they are not. The pleasure of eating the unhealthy food is stronger than the perceived pain of not being able to have it. We always move toward pleasure and away from pain. One day, this person has a heart attack, and the very next day they begin to follow all the healthy recommendations they were avoiding before, with great resolve. Their whole outlook and motivation on diet and health has turned 180 degrees. What has changed? Why is this person now able to eat completely differently with ease and without struggle? Having the heart attack changed how they look at eating healthy and the thoughts they now have around their diet. Their previous thoughts of "eating healthy is boring and tastes bad; I don't like fruits and vegetables; I can't enjoy my food unless it's loaded with sugar or is fried," lead to an inaction of eating healthy food. After having the heart attack, their thoughts turned into "making healthy choices will help me lead a life of quality; I will see my kids get married and have a chance to play with my grandchildren." This in turn produced feelings of motivation and determination which they were then able to take action on, so that eating healthy was in direct harmony with their thoughts and feelings.

Another example is overeating: whether it is finishing the bag of chips after you have told yourself you won't have any, or eating two slices of cake even though you are full—whatever it may be for you— the action is eating the food. Working backward, what are the feelings you are experiencing when you are eating the food? It may be that you are feeling anxious or bored, unhappy or frustrated, or have self-loathing. Those feelings are leading you to overeat. Let's look even further back. What are the thoughts you are having that are leading to those feelings? Are you thinking about your stress at work that is giving you the feeling of anxiety? Are you focusing on the fight you had with your spouse? Are you thinking that there is no point in trying to lose weight, and that it will never work? Just sit with this information for a while and look at it from an inquisitive point of view. Really take a step back and be curious without any judgment or being defensive, and look at yourself with compassion and love. You have formed a pattern and a connection with those thoughts and feelings and food. And our mind loves patterns: doing the same thing over and over. So, now it has become a habit where your thoughts about work, or your dissatisfaction with your relationship or with losing weight, produce feelings that lead you to overeat.

Once you understand this, you can then decide if you want to change this pattern by changing your thoughts.

Change your thoughts before taking action to avoid the struggle between what you "should" do, and your feelings about it.

I see it, I feel it, I have it

You often hear about competitive athletes visualizing being successful—scoring that goal, landing that jump, or winning that final game. The reason visualization works in helping you reach your goals is because your Unconscious Mind does not distinguish between real and imagined events, especially when accompanied by strong emotion.

Read through the following paragraph first and then imagine it or record it, and play it back to yourself:

Close your eyes and imagine you are lying on a hammock on the beach with a slight breeze blowing, as you are listening to the calming sound the ocean waves make as they flow toward the shore. The birds are quietly chirping in the background as your hammock sways slowly from side to side. You are filled with gratitude and a sense of calm and you are basking in the warm rays of the sun.

Now open your eyes. How do you feel? Did you feel like you were in the hammock? Are you now filled with a sense of calm? Your actual physical environment of where you are right now, reading this book, has not changed, yet how you are feeling may have.

You can feel the exact same emotions from something that is actually happening or something you are only thinking about. Have you ever watched a movie that made you cry? Maybe it was a love story, like *The Notebook,* where rich girl Allie's first love returns after the war and, even though she is involved with another man, it is obvious that their love is still strong. I know I cried watching this movie, the whole time knowing full well that it was just a movie with actors acting out their scenes. The same thing happens when you use your imagination to visualize. It takes on the imagination as if it is real.

Your Unconscious Mind is always listening to what you are saying, and it is watching everything you do. It is not emotional and it is there to protect you; that's why it acts on your self-limiting beliefs. It thinks that is what you want. You can help override your unconscious self-limiting beliefs that are sabotaging your success. Visualization with positive thoughts and positive emotion will help to convince your Unconscious Mind that what you are saying you want consciously, is what you really want and will help to align your CM's and your UM's desires. The more you visualize, the more your Private Detective (RAS) will work to bring you what you need to be successful.

This does not mean you can sit back and do nothing. You are still responsible for the change you want to achieve. What *will* become possible, is that you will no longer be your own saboteur. If you are focusing on, and visualizing, that having a healthy body is what you want, and you put positive feeling into it, your Unconscious Mind will listen. On the other hand, if you say to yourself that eating healthy and participating in any physical activity is too difficult, your Unconscious Mind will think of working toward your goal as an unpleasant experience and will do everything so that you don't feel that unpleasantness. Remember, we tend to move toward pleasure and away from pain. If you are saying to yourself how good it feels to take care of your body, to move it regularly, to try new healthy recipes, your Unconscious Mind will help you take action on those behaviours that support it. The key is to imagine the experience in a positive, energizing, motivating way. Put lots of positive feeling into it!

> ***You can feel the exact same emotions from something that is real or imagined.***

Does replacing your limiting beliefs guarantee you will automatically have the body you want? Not exactly, but it *will* make it possible for you to take action toward your success by choosing foods which will help you reach your goal of being healthy, being at a healthy weight, becoming more active, and eating according to your hunger. Imagine eating food that will give you the nourishment that your body requires and deserves! Imagine eating when you are hungry and stopping when you are full. Imagine what it would be like to have control over eating chips or pizza or cake, and being able to stop before eating all of it? Imagine eating without guilt and without judgment coming from inside your head. This is all possible when you let go of your limiting beliefs that are keeping you stuck in your problem.

Every morning, and often throughout the day, visualize the image of yourself being slim, healthy, and strongly motivated, and feeling happy and excited!

Now that I have shown you how to take your power back from the Mean Girl, and the importance of your thoughts in producing the action you want, it's time to look at what is missing in your life and how to set boundaries.

Chapter 5

What's Missing?

Why Can't I Say "NO?"

Have you ever been asked to do something and, without thinking, you said *YES*, when you actually wanted to say *NO*? Requests are made of us on a daily basis. You would think that by now we would have enough practice at dealing with them to be able to respond with how we really feel. When was the last time a request was made of you and you automatically said *YES*? This may have happened at work when your boss placed another project on your desk even though your pile of work was already unbearable; or perhaps at home when your husband asked if your in-laws could come for dinner on the weekend when you were looking forward to just relaxing? Can you recall the last time you answered the opposite of what you really wanted to say? What feelings were you experiencing as you continued to berate yourself for saying yes? Did you get angry at yourself? What about toward the person who you said *YES* to? Did you start to feel resentment toward them? What kind of feelings were you experiencing every time you replayed the scenario in your head? Why is it that we, women in particular, have such a hard time saying *NO*?

Part of it has to do with what we discussed earlier, being the Driver vs the Passenger. If you are constantly feeling like you are a victim, being pushed around by other people and being taken advantage of, well, you are still the Passenger. You do not think you have control over what is thrown at you. Think about people who are successful. What kind of attitude do you think they have in life? If they are acting like pushovers, how far will that take them toward their goals?

Consider why you might say *YES* when you want to say *NO*. Are you afraid of not being liked? Are you a "people pleaser?" Do you put your needs last on the list? Do you believe that saying *YES* when you mean *NO* is helpful to the person asking something of you? Let's look at this scenario from a client of mine.

Deborah T.

Deborah T. decided to get back into the workforce once her children started school and she was not required to be home during the day. She chose a Direct Sales position, selling make-up through in-home parties. She believed that a great way to get clients and get her name out there was to attend networking events in her area. These events were usually once a month in the evening, and she would require her husband to be home to get dinner ready and stay with the kids. Deborah looked forward to these events as it was a way to get out of the house, meet new and interesting women, and potential clients.

On the day of one of the events, Deborah had picked out her outfit and made sure that she had lots of business cards ready, as well as catalogues, to show off the products she was selling. That evening, 2 hours before Deborah's event, her husband called her to say that he was going out for dinner and drinks with his buddies after work. Deborah's reply was, "OK," even though she was not OK with it. This meant that she could not attend her networking event and had to stay home with the kids. As she continued to replay the conversation in her head, her resentment toward her husband grew. "He always gets to do whatever he wants and I get stuck at home. This is so unfair," were some of the thoughts running through her head. Her husband was, of course, oblivious to what was going through Deborah's head, because this conversation was happening *in her head*. When Deborah's husband came home later in the evening, Deborah was barely talking to him and giving him the cold shoulder. When he asked her if anything was the matter, Deborah's reply was, "Nothing." Deborah's husband assumed that Deborah was just tired or was frustrated with one of the children, and then forgot about it.

If Deborah continues to keep quiet about her needs, her resentment toward her husband will increase and it will affect their relationship.

If you say *YES* when you mean *NO*, you are letting another person be responsible for and lead your life. You are saying that it is OK for other people to make decisions for you. You are behaving as a Passenger in your own life. Think about all the times in your life where you give your control to others.

It is important to set boundaries in your life when it comes to other people and their demands. Saying how you really feel means getting control back into your life and sitting in the Driver's seat. This is how you communicate your feelings, and your needs and wants, to another person. Women too often expect others to read their mind and, when that doesn't happen, resentment sets in.

Just like boundaries between countries that objectively state where one country ends and another begins, so should your personal/ emotional/physical boundaries. It is simply a limit beyond which you will not feel happy, safe, respected, or fulfilled. When these limits are stated clearly, the person making the request has specific parameters to work with. This is required for a healthy relationship. Anytime you feel resentful or unhappy by saying YES, it is an indication that your limit was crossed. Keep in mind that it was crossed because you did not communicate to the other person what your needs and wants are.

> **Saying YES when you want to say NO is unhealthy for any relationship you have.**

If you are afraid to say *NO* because you feel you will not be seen as a nice person, and then become resentful and hold a grudge toward your spouse, mother, or boss, in actuality, this is what makes you a "not nice" person. Keeping this information from another person denies them the chance to act in the way that you require. This is a very passive-aggressive way to behave and can hurt a relationship.

You may feel that allowing a member of your family to get their way will keep peace in the family. Your mother-in-law showing up unannounced might make your blood curdle when you are in the midst of helping your kids with homework while simultaneously cooking dinner, yet you say nothing about how you would like her to call before she wants to come over to see if it's a good time. This is not only unfair to you, but it is also unfair to your mother-in-law. She may be thinking that she is helping you when she comes over, and has no idea about how you really feel.

If you allow your spouse to make all the decisions because you don't want to stir the pot, and are afraid to get into conflict, he will continue to bypass you on your opinion. The longer you allow others to be the Driver of your life, the harder it will be to get back into the Driver's seat. How much longer will you allow yourself to feel powerless? Isn't it time you moved yourself into a powerful mindset?

The good news is that it is never too late to become the Driver of your life. It's never too late to start setting limits and boundaries. How you set your boundaries is important. Stating what you want clearly does not mean that you don't care about the person asking something of you. It is showing that person how to respect you and will make it easier for them to know what is expected. Coming at your spouse with blame for all the times in the past when he came home late after an evening with the boys, will not put him into a mindset to listen to what you have to say. Put your feelings of blame and resentment aside.

If you quickly answer YES to a request, without thinking and then regret it later, the first step is taking a PAUSE. The request may be of you giving your time, or it may be for money or for your energy. If your sister-in-law calls you and asks if she can drop off her 3 kids on Saturday for you to take care of, and your usual go to answer is *YES*, even though it makes you feel resentful because Saturday is your only day off—take a pause. You can tell her that you need to check your schedule and will get back to her later in the evening. Taking a pause will allow you to really decide how you feel about the request and your response. During the pause, decide whether you have the following 3 things: the time to fulfill the request, the desire to fulfill the request and, lastly, the cash (if applicable) to fulfill the request. In your sister-in-law's case, she is asking of your time and your desire. If the answer to both of those is *NO*, then when you call her back, say, "I will not be able to watch your kids this Saturday; this is the only day I have to get my stuff done." End of story. If on the other hand, you do have time available, and you are happy to see your niece and nephew, decide how you can say *YES* to your sister-in-law and still feel you are not being taken advantage of. Perhaps you are happy to go to her house where the kids have their toys, and stay with the kids there for 3 hours. Or maybe you want to take them out for lunch and give your sister-in-law a break for a couple of hours. You can modify the request in a way so that it is on your terms.

THE STEPS:
1. PAUSE
2. DECIDE
3. MODIFY
4. SPEAK

Let's get back to Deborah T. who told her husband it was okay to go see his buddies even though it meant she missed her monthly networking event. We strategized on what Deborah could have done instead. When her husband called her, Deborah could have taken the necessary pause before answering by saying she would call him back in a few minutes. During this pause, Deborah could have then decided the following: did she have the time to stay at home this evening so her husband could go out for dinner and drinks? The answer was *NO*. The networking event was important for Deborah to build her business. Was there a way to modify the request and still be able to go to the networking event? Deborah came up with a modification. She called her husband back and stated the following: You will have to come home from work so that I can attend my networking event, which you know is important to me to grow my business. I will have dinner prepared and the kids will be washed and ready for bed. I will come home after the event and you will still be able to join your friends for after dinner drinks.

The last important step in setting your boundary is that you may need to have a consequence for the person you are setting it for, if your boundary is not respected. This is not to punish the other person but to allow them to see that this boundary is very important to you and you are serious about it. When you set a boundary, the other person is not obliged to follow it. It's nice if they do, but you can't make them. Setting a consequence and communicating it with the person, lets them know what to expect if they do not respect your limit.

Getting back to the example of your mother-in-law showing up unannounced, you can explain to her that although you love that she spends time with her grandchildren, she needs to call before she wants to come to make sure it is an appropriate time. If she does not call and comes unannounced, you can let her know that you won't be able to let her inside the house as it may not be a good time.

It may feel scary to be so assertive when speaking. Remember that you are showing people how to treat you. Begin to practice boundary setting with small matters and requests and, as you get more confident, work your way up to bigger matters. Write down daily in a journal how you responded to a request that was made of you. Remember the steps plus the consequence. This may take practice, especially if you are a people pleaser and have been allowing other people to be the Driver of your life.

A small request could come from your teenager asking you to wash her favourite shirt at 11 o'clock at night for the next morning. You can set a boundary that you will wash her clothes if they are brought to the laundry room ahead of time, and she needs to let you know by 5 pm if there is something there that needs to be washed "urgently." Her consequence is that if she does not let you know in advance and does not bring her laundry to the laundry room, the clothes will not be washed. It is imperative that you stick to the consequence you have set, or else your boundary will not be respected.

> ***Setting boundaries will put you in the Driver's seat of your life.***

From Blah to Wow

Life can be busy and chaotic. Sometimes in the midst of doing the day-to-day chores, working, having hectic schedules, being a taxi driver for the kids, and doing never-ending laundry, you forget to focus on *YOU*. Often women put everyone and everything above their own needs and wants. You may know and feel that you are unhappy, unmotivated, apathetic, and are generally going through the motions of life, but you are so busy with the "motions" that you never give your needs a second thought. So what do you do to make yourself feel better? You grab that bag of chips waiting for you in your pantry. How often do you think about *your* needs and wants? How often do you do something for yourself—for your spiritual, physical, or mental health? Do you feel guilty after you take time out for yourself because that other "to do" list is waiting for you? Let's delve a little deeper into "The Life of You," and see if you are taking care of yourself and your needs or if you are just an afterthought.

You will discover how fulfilled you are in different areas of your life and what you can do to go from BLAH to WOW! Below is your life divided into 9 segments, and for each segment I want you to rate how fulfilled you are with that area of your life, ranging from 0 (completely unfulfilled) to 10 (completely fulfilled). For a free, print-ready download of this worksheet, go to www.ItsNotAboutTheCheesecake .com.

Career/Job

0   1   2   3   4   5   6   7   8   9   10

Finances/Money

0   1   2   3   4   5   6   7   8   9   10

Love/Romance

0   1   2   3   4   5   6   7   8   9   10

Health

0   1   2   3   4   5   6   7   8   9   10

Family

0   1   2   3   4   5   6   7   8   9   10

Relationships

0   1   2   3   4   5   6   7   8   9   10

Fun/Social Life

0   1   2   3   4   5   6   7   8   9   10

Me time

0   1   2   3   4   5   6   7   8   9   10

Personal Growth

0   1   2   3   4   5   6   7   8   9   10

Circle the areas in your life where your satisfaction score is 6 or less. How do you deal with being less fulfilled in these areas? What is your coping mechanism? Are you using food to help yourself feel better about not having the life you want? Do you overeat so you don't have to feel your unhappiness? Are you numbing your feelings with food? Food can only satisfy a physical hunger. No amount or type of food will satisfy emotional hunger or make you feel more fulfilled in your life.

From the list, choose your life segments where you scored 6 or less and answer the following: For a free, full size, print-ready download of this worksheet, go to www.ItsNotAboutTheCheesecake.com.

1. What do you do now to make yourself feel better in this area of your life, or when you have a problem in this area?

2. How satisfied are you in how you deal with it?

Career/Job

_____

_____

_____

Finances/Money

_____
_____
_____

Love/Romance

_____
_____
_____

Health

_____
_____
_____

Family

_____
_____
_____

Relationships

_____
_____
_____

Fun/SociaLife

_____
_____
_____

Me Time

_____
_____
_____

Personal Growth

_____

_____

_____

> ***Food can never satisfy an emotional need.***

Having completed the list, what did you discover? How many parts of your life are you unfulfilled in? Are you surprised by the number? How are you currently managing the fact that something is lacking in that area of your life? Are you trying your best to ignore it? Or are you using food as a management technique to make yourself feel better?

Monica B.

When Monica B. stepped into my office, the first words out of her mouth were, "My problem is that I just love food too much." She explained her hectic life with 3 kids and their extra-curricular activities, taking care of her husband, and taking care of the house. Between driving her kids to and from school, bringing them to their various after-school programs, preparing all of the meals and the laundry and cleaning, the only time she felt she could relax and unwind was after the kids went to bed, the kitchen was clean, and lunches were prepared for the next day. That quiet time in the evening was her personal time, and she would raid the kitchen, especially the cupboard where she kept all those snacks "for the kids," and sit in front of the TV and eat. She consumed large amounts of calories, eating until she felt so stuffed she could hardly move. She would then hide all of the wrappers at the bottom of the garbage, so her husband would not find out, and head to bed.

The results of Monica's life satisfaction exercise revealed that her score for Love and Romance was a 3, her score for Relationship was a 4, and her score for Fun was a 2. When we explored those areas of her life further, it became clear that instead of focusing on those areas and doing something to become more fulfilled to make her score higher, Monica was turning to food for fulfillment. Food had become the most meaningful and purposeful part of her day. Turning to food did nothing to increase her joy and satisfaction in those areas of her life. In fact, as her weight increased, she felt more and more dissatisfied with herself and life.

Go back to your results and decide what you can do to improve your satisfaction score in your low satisfaction areas—something that does not involve food. What will you do instead of eating? What can you do that will bring you closer to your goal in that area of your life?
We explored what Monica could do instead of eating to increase her happiness in the 3 areas where she scored low. Using food as a solution was not taking her closer to happiness and she realized that. She decided that she would ask her Mom to babysit on Friday evenings so that she and her husband could have "date night" and begin to communicate again. Her Mom readily agreed and, when she brought up the idea to her husband, he was elated.

It is possible that the people around you do not necessarily share the same wants as you do. Perhaps your spouse is not interested in spending date night with you. You can still improve your life satisfaction score—just focus on YOU! If you score low in the FUN category, perhaps a weekly evening out with your girlfriends will bring your score higher. You are the Driver of your life and you get to decide what you need to satisfy your needs and wants.

Now you know why setting boundaries and getting your life needs met are so important to your success! In the next chapter, let's explore the different types of hunger, how to know if you are actually hungry, why you may need to eat your trigger foods, and how you can eliminate your cravings.

Chapter 6

Remember To Eat

The Forgotten Hunger

Have you ever watched a baby being fed? When the baby is hungry, everyone in the room will know; he will get more and more agitated and his cries will get louder and louder until he is given nourishment. What happens after he has had enough? He becomes completely disinterested in food, turns his head away, and may purse his lips or start to spit. It's very difficult to feed a baby who is not hungry. In fact, when parents ignore a baby's internal cues for hunger and fullness, and try to force food into his mouth, they are teaching him to disregard his internal signals and, if this practice continues, are setting him up for an unhealthy relationship with food. Babies intrinsically know when they are hungry and when they've had enough. They follow their physical cues.

How often do you eat when you are not hungry? Do you wait for the hunger cues before eating? Do you stop eating when you are satisfied, or do you clean off your plate even if you've had enough? Eating for emotional reasons is very different than eating because you are physically hungry. The section below distinguishes between physical and emotional hunger. Are you able to get in touch with hunger and fullness signals in your body?

PHYSICAL HUNGER

- Comes on gradually and you can wait to eat

- Hunger is felt in the stomach: rumbling, feeling of emptiness

- Can be satisfied with many different foods

- You stop when you are comfortably full

- After eating, you feel satisfied and have no bad feelings about yourself

EMOTIONAL HUNGER

- Comes on suddenly and has a sense of urgency

- Hunger is felt "above the neck." Your mind is swirling with thoughts about the food. Craving for the food is felt in the mouth and the mind

- Only satisfied with specific foods (chocolate, pizza, chips, ice-cream, fast-food)

- You ignore satiety cues and eat until you are uncomfortably full

- After eating, you feel badly about yourself (shame, guilt, worthlessness)

Adapted from: *Constant Craving: What Your Food Cravings Mean and How to Overcome Them* By Doreen Virtue, PhD, published by Hay House, Inc., 1995

Paying attention to your body will help you get in touch with feelings of true physical hunger. This may prove to be difficult at first because years of dieting and chaotic eating patterns may have allowed you to lose touch with the physical signals. You may have ignored them for so long that you don't pay attention to them anymore. If your eating pattern is to eat all day long with no breaks, then you never allow yourself to get hungry and may not remember what that feels like.

The best place to start is with a structured schedule for meal time, which will allow time in between for your body to become physically hungry. Your day should start with eating breakfast within 1–2 hours of waking, and then eat approximately every 3–4 hours after that. Use the Hunger Scale below to help you become aware of your physical hunger. For a free, pocket size, print ready copy, go to www.ItsNot AboutTheCheesecake.com.

THE HUNGER SCALE

1   Starving, shaky, lightheaded, weak

2   Very hungry, poor concentration

3   Hungry, stomach rumbling, can eat a meal

4   Slightly hungry, can eat a snack

5   Neutral, not hungry and not full

6   Slightly full, can still eat some more

7   Satisfied and comfortably full

8   Full

9   Uncomfortably full

10 Stuffed, feeling sick, nauseous

Become aware of where you are on the scale whenever you eat, as well as when you finish eating. When you are at a 3–4, and are experiencing comfortable signs of physical hunger, you should eat. Choose foods that will satisfy you—what your body wants and what your body needs. Once you reach a 6–7 on the hunger scale, it is time for you to stop eating. When you diet, you try to overpower your natural hunger and satiety signals, which is an unnatural way to eat. You are also relying only on external cues to tell you when you should eat or have had enough, instead of internal cues. As you have likely experienced, restricted types of eating will only lead to bingeing and more disordered eating. Eating to your hunger and fullness cues is a natural way to eat.

You might be thinking that if you are "allowed" to eat anything you want, you will lose control over your eating and only eat foods that are unhealthy and full of fat, salt, and sugar. Likely, when you are "pigging out" on these foods, it is either because you are using food to satisfy an emotional need, because you have been depriving yourself so strictly from these foods, or you have "all or nothing thinking" (e.g., I'm going to overeat this cake because, from tomorrow on, I am on a strict diet and cannot ever have cake.). Following the hunger scale will actually give you more control around food and meals. You do not have to be consumed with thoughts regarding what you can or cannot eat. No food is forbidden. Follow the principles in the next section to help you.

> ***Eat when you are hungry and stop when you are comfortably full.***

From Mindless to Mindful

When was the last time you ate a meal and really enjoyed it from beginning to end? I mean, really savoured every single bite? Did you enjoy every morsel because it was so good, or just ate it because it was there in front of you? We often eat without really paying attention to what is in front of us. If you eat in front of the TV, then you are more engrossed in your show than the food. The food travelling into your mouth becomes an automatic activity. Do you finish the food from your kids' plates that they've left after a meal? Ask yourself why. In the previous section I discussed hunger and satiety cues. When you begin to eat off of your kids' plates, what number is your hunger at? Do you even pay attention?

I used to mindlessly eat in the car. I would stop at a grocery store, head straight for their bakery section, and buy a few pastries—3 or 4 regular sized pastries, not the mini ones. Of course, I always asked the person behind the counter to put it nicely in a box to make it seem that I was taking the pastries to be shared amongst a few people. I would then rush back to the car and start devouring what I had just bought. I didn't stop until the box was empty. It felt like I didn't even breathe until I had finished the entire box of pastries, or I got so sick from all the sugar and fat I had just ingested that I became nauseous. The empty box or the nausea was my only sign to stop.

Mindless eating is when you are eating without awareness to your hunger and satiety cues, or to what and how much you are consuming. Eating mindlessly is not pleasurable, it is done as if you are on auto-pilot, without thought or reasoning and without control. Eating mindlessly is driven by emotions and not paying attention to your body's physical signals. *Mindful eating*, on the other hand, is the exact opposite: it is eating in coordination with your body's cues to hunger and satiety, actually tasting and enjoying the food you are eating, being in the present, and being aware of your surroundings.

Think back to the last time you were at a restaurant and ordered a big bowl of pasta (Some portions are large enough to feed a whole family!). You likely really enjoyed the first few forkfuls; you may have been hungry and even the thought of the upcoming dish got you salivating. By the time you were half way done with the dish, did you even notice what you were eating? Likely not. When we are presented with food that we like, we really enjoy the first few bites because we were so looking forward to it; we may even enjoy the last couple of bites because we know that afterwards the bowl will be empty and there will be no more—the middle bites are just fillers. Once we have satisfied our hunger, and our taste buds get used to the taste of what we are eating, we don't even notice the food anymore until the very end. We are consuming all these excess calories without deriving any pleasure from it!

> *We enjoy the first few bites*
> *and the last few bites of our food.*

Here are some strategies to use to make sure you are eating Mindfully:

1. Eat according to your hunger

How hungry are you? Look back on the previous section where I discussed the Hunger Scale. Check-in with yourself where you are on the scale before eating. Remember that eating for anything other than physical hunger will not satisfy your emotional needs. When you are between 3–4 on the scale, go ahead and eat. If you are lower on the Hunger Scale, at a 1 or 2, you are likely starving and have missed the best window of when to eat, and it may be more difficult for you to eat mindfully. Use this as feedback that you may have gone too long without eating or not eaten enough the meal before. Any higher number than 4 on the scale means you are not yet hungry enough to eat and may want food for other reasons.

2. Eat slowly

Ever hear the old saying that it takes 20 minutes for your brain to realize you are full? A feeling of fullness is only one signal that you have had enough to eat; the brain also receives signals from digestive hormones. When you eat too quickly, you are way ahead of your satiety signals and, by the time they kick in, you are well on your way to finishing dessert. Eating slowly allows you to know when you have had enough. You can slow down your eating by putting your cutlery back down on your plate between mouthfuls. Make sure you have chewed and swallowed the food before you once again pick up your fork or spoon. Chewing the food well is very important because digestion starts in the mouth, and this will also help you avoid unnecessary indigestion, bloating, and heartburn. If you are in a group setting, see who the slower eater is and mimic them. Stop eating half way through your meal and ask yourself where you are on the Hunger Scale. If you are at 6–7, you are full enough; any extra bites will not be mindful. If you are still at 4 –5, continue eating.

3. Eat what you desire

Instead of putting strict limitations on what you "should" and "should not eat," which only increases the desire for the foods you "should not" eat, eat what you actually want. Depriving yourself of certain foods makes them more appealing. Let's say I tell you to never eat chocolate chip cookies again; you are now going to be thinking about chocolate chip cookies all the time. Your Reticular Activating System will be picking out all the bakeries on your way to work that sell cookies. You will begin to have cravings for chocolate chip cookies like never before. Deprivation leads to bingeing. Have you ever had a craving for a food, and tried to overcome that craving by eating something else? How did that work for you? Did you find that you kept searching for and eating foods that you were "supposed to eat," only to succumb to your craving and still eat that forbidden food? You may be concerned that if you don't put any restrictions on what you are "allowed" to eat, you will only eat high fat, high sugar foods and gain even more weight! Remember, you are eating to satisfy your physical hunger, not your emotional hunger. When you eat with the knowledge that this food will be there tomorrow and the day after, you stop eating out of restriction and fear. Mindful eating is eating without judgment about yourself.

4. Taste and Savour

Speed eating and eating on automatic pilot deprives your senses of actually enjoying, tasting, and celebrating the food. Taking time to see, smell, taste, and swallow the food will give you a new appreciation for what you are eating.

Do the following exercise with a fresh berry or a nut, or dried fruit or any other small piece of food you have on hand. The point of this exercise is to use as many of your senses as possible.

Look at the food:

Take a close look at the piece of food you have chosen. Look at the colour, the shape, and texture.

Smell the food:

Bring the food close to your nose and really take in the fragrance. Does it bring out any emotion or any memories? How does the smell make you feel?

Taste the food (do this with your eyes closed):

Put the piece of food in your mouth, but don't bite it. Roll it around in your mouth and really feel the texture of it.

Take one bite:

As you bite the food, what are the sensations? Is it hard? Soft? Juicy? Grainy? Smooth?

Chew the food:

Notice what is happening to the texture of the food. Notice the explosion of taste in your mouth. Notice the intensity of the flavour changing the more you chew. Continue slowly chewing at least 10 more times.

Swallow the food:

As you swallow the food, focus on the sensation of it as it travels down your throat.

Although these steps are somewhat exaggerated, this will help you focus on your sensory experience of eating.

5. Eat to your fullness

Stop eating when you are at 6–7 on the Hunger Scale. There is no urgent need to finish all of the food because you can have it any time you like. You are not starting a diet tomorrow; therefore, you do not need to eat as much as you can today. We often rely on external signals to let us know when the meal is done, such as an empty plate or if it's time to get back to work after your lunch hour. Look for internal signals of when to finish a meal: hungry or full; thirsty or satisfied. If you always finish everything on your plate, start leaving a little bit of food, even if it's a forkful; at the same time, listen to your satiety cues. This will help to program your mind that it is ok to leave food on the plate.

6. Eat at the table

Eating at the table will help you to focus on what and how much you are eating without distractions. Make sure the TV is off if you have one in the kitchen. If you consistently eat all meals and snacks at the table, you will be less likely to eat on auto-pilot. Don't multi-task during meals.

Some people like to snack while watching TV, out of habit. Having all of your meals and snacks in the kitchen will help you break that habit. If you feel that you need to do something with your hands because you are so used to eating while watching TV, try solving a Rubik's Cube, or take up knitting or pet your dog.

Does following these principles mean you will never again eat until you are uncomfortably stuffed or wait too long to have a meal? Not at all. But it does mean that you are now aware of why you are eating and why you may be overeating. Just remind yourself of the principles and return to eating mindfully. To help you with your awareness, keep a daily food journal to record where you are on your hunger scale when you started and when you stopped the meal or snack, as well as any thoughts and feelings you have just before, during, or right after the meal. For a free, full size print-ready download of this worksheet go to www.ItsNotAboutTheCheesecake.com.

MEAL/TIME	FOOD and AMOUNT	HUNGER SCALE 1 starving-10 stuffed	FEELINGS, SELF-TALK

Food – Friend or Foe?

When you think about food, what types of thoughts and feelings pop into your head? Does food make you feel like you have no control? Do you feel powerless when your trigger foods are placed in front of you? Or do you feel that food is your loyal friend, and is always there to comfort you? All of these feelings are very common to my clients. They personalize their relationship with food as if food has feelings, and will reciprocate the feelings they have toward it. Some feel that food is the enemy and is out to hurt them and make their life miserable. Does this sound like you? Food is neither good nor bad. It is neither your friend nor your enemy. It doesn't care if you are having a bad day, or just broke up with your boyfriend or got that job promotion. By personalizing your relationship to food and giving this relationship meaning and emotions, you are allowing the food to have power over you. Guess what? Food doesn't care; it is just there.

Some of the emotional attachment to food that you have now, you may have linked since childhood. The food may represent a relationship experience. Perhaps when you were a child, your grandmother would bake delicious cakes that you and your family enjoyed. So cake now has the emotional experiences of your childhood attached to it. Now every time you see and eat cake, all of those good emotions of spending time with your grandmother are felt along with eating the food. Not only do you enjoy the taste of the cake, but you also enjoy the emotional experience that goes along with it. Or, perhaps, popcorn reminds you of the times you had "movie nights" with your family and would make big bowls of extra buttery popcorn. Now, when you have popcorn in front of you, you don't stop eating until the bag is empty.

Keeping these trigger foods away from your home or office is more of a band-aid approach that will not last forever. This tactic will work as long as you have complete control over your environment. However, as we all know, you can't always have control over your environment. Yes, you can refrain from buying chips and bringing them home but, inevitably, you will go to a party or a friend's house, and the chips will be there. By now you know that willpower is not the answer, because there is no such thing.

The solution is to prescribe that food as part of your eating regime. By eating your trigger foods on your terms, the food will no longer have power over you. Make a decision when and how much of that food you will have, keeping in mind the mindful way of eating discussed earlier in this chapter. If carrot cake is your trigger food, you may want to decide that on Friday nights when you go out with your girlfriends, you will share a slice of cake. This frees up your time, all the other days, to focus on your goals without feeling deprivation. Remember that deprivation will only lead to bingeing and feeling out of control. It can only work in the short term, and will leave you feeling even worse in the long term.

List your trigger food(s):

_____
_____
_____

Decide how you will you incorporate these foods as part of your eating pattern

_____
_____
_____
_____

What food has emotional forces for you?

When I eat _____
I feel_____

Example: When I eat cake, I feel calm.

How can I satisfy these emotional needs other than with food (e.g., meet up with a friend, spend time with my children, volunteer, etc.)?

_____
_____
_____
_____

Pizza and Chocolate and Chips, Oh My!

As you are successfully combatting your inner negative self-talk and eating with more awareness of your physical hunger and fullness, you may still have that one particular food that you feel has power over you. Perhaps it's donuts or chips, or chocolate covered almonds; whatever it may be, when that food is put in front of you, you feel out of control. For me, it was mini cheese danishes at a bakery across from my kids' school. I would sit in my car in the parking lot in front of the bakery waiting for my kids to come out from their classes at the end of the day. The smell of freshly baked bread and delicious sweets made my mouth water. I would go into the bakery and promptly buy 5 or 6 mini danishes to eat in my car while waiting for my kids. The only control I had was seeing the bag of danishes empty. That was my clue to stop. Those danishes were completely controlling me—that is until I learned a powerful technique that I'm going to share with you. It takes moments to learn and will help you get control over a particular craving. Keep in mind, you were not born craving pizza, just as I was not born craving danishes. This is a completely learned behaviour which can be unlearned.

Have you ever had food poisoning after you had eaten a particular food, and from that moment can't even stand the thought of that food, let alone eat it? Your brain became wired to respond a particular way toward this food. The food hasn't changed, but the way you feel about it has. I remember when I was pregnant with my daughter; I was very nauseous the first 3 months. One day I was eating a bowl of pineapple and then became so nauseous that I ended up vomiting soon after. Since then, I cannot even think about pineapple without getting a nauseated feeling in my stomach and throat.

You can use the Craving Terminator technique below to rewire your brain to no longer think of pleasure that is currently associated with the food. You will see the power that imagination and your mind can have in getting exactly what you want, since the brain does not distinguish the difference between a real experience and a vividly imagined one.

Craving Terminator[2]

This technique will result in your not wanting to eat a particular food ever again. Before you continue with reading and then doing the technique, make sure that you are truly okay with banishing the desire you have for this food.

Pick a food you want to stop craving. It has to be very specific. For example, if your food is "chips," pick a specific flavour and brand of chips. For me it was the mini cheese danishes made in the bakery across from the school.

Make sure you read through all of the steps first before doing the exercise.

1. Imagine that the food you want to stop craving is in front of you. Remember to be specific. Is it in a bowl or on a plate, or in a bag? See the food and all of the sensations that come with having it in front of you. Imagine the smell, texture, and taste as you are putting it into your mouth. Make the picture vivid and real.

2. Now think of something that would be repulsive to you if you saw it in front of you on a plate. Something that is utterly disgusting and gross. For me it is a plate full of crawling maggots. It may be a plate full of hair or cockroaches, or dog excrement.

3. I want you to imagine a plate full of whatever it is you are repulsed by (from #2) in front of you. Look closely into the plate. Imagine

---

[2] Adapted from Paul McKenna, *I Can Make You Thin* (Toronto, Canada by Sterling Publishing 2009) 126.

smelling and licking whatever it is that you chose that's on your plate. As you are imagining this, squeeze your right earlobe with your thumb and finger. Continue to imagine yourself eating whatever is on your plate, putting it into your mouth and rolling it with your tongue, really feeling the texture of it. Continue to squeeze your earlobe together as you imagine this, as you are feeling completely disgusted and sick.

Break the image in your head by imagining a white screen for a few seconds and letting go of your earlobe. Repeat #3 at least four more times, each time squeezing your right earlobe as you think about the repulsive item and then letting go of the earlobe and clearing the image with a white screen for a few seconds.

4. Next, imagine the food you want to stop craving (e.g., mini danishes). Imagine it is in front of you on a plate or in a bowl. Now, imagine it mixed with the repulsive item from #2 (e.g., crawling maggots). Really mix up your favourite food with the repulsive items in the plate, until you can no longer imagine your favourite food without combining it with the repulsive item. They are completely mixed on the plate. Imagine eating both of those items together; you are tasting some of your favourite food and it is mixed with the texture, smell, and taste of the item you are repulsed by. As you do this, squeeze your right earlobe.

Clear your thought by imagining a white screen and let go of your earlobe. Repeat #4 four more times, each time imagining the taste and smell getting worse and worse as you are eating and swallowing the two items. Continue to do this until you are utterly disgusted when you imagine having these items combined together.

5. Now imagine a gigantic glob of this disgusting food is in front of you (e.g., mini danishes mixed with maggots). In a moment, you are going to imagine it coming at you at lightning speed. It's going

to go through you with all the revolting feeling and smell, and with a screeching sound. It will move right through you, and you will sense it behind you on the count of three. Ready? 1, 2, 3, WOOSH!

6. Think about that food you're used to have a craving for, and notice how you feel about it now.

Repeat all of the steps at least 5 times or until your craving is completely gone.

Now that you have learned how to listen to your internal cues of when it's time to eat and when it's time to stop eating, and how to truly enjoy all foods, it is time to get motivated and set some goals!

Chapter 7

Having It All

The Motivator Technique

How would you like to replace a negative behavior that is keeping you stuck, with a positive one that will help you move toward your goal? By now, you know that your thoughts lead to feelings, which lead to a behavior or an action. Positive thoughts will produce positive actions that will guide you toward your goal, and negative thoughts will produce negative feelings that will produce a negative action (or a lack of an action) that will take you further from your goal. If your thoughts about exercise are that it is boring and difficult, the resulting feelings will be procrastination, apathy, and a lack of motivation. This will lead to an inaction. (You will be less likely to engage in physical activity.)

The Motivator Technique[3] will not only help you get rid of the negative feelings and action (or lack of action) that is not serving you well, but it will also replace those negative feelings with positive ones which will lead to a positive action. In fact, these positive feelings will become automatic! You will no longer be in a tug of war between what you consciously want and how you feel unconsciously.

Let's look at the example of not engaging in physical activity. You may have formed a pattern in your mind which starts with your negative

---

[3] Adapted from Joseph McClendon III, *STOP IT Method,* 2016

thoughts in relation to being active, followed by a negative emotion. In the technique below, your first step will be to feel the negative emotion that you want to change, so you can then disrupt it and swap it. You will then break that pattern of emotion so that it can be replaced with the opposite emotion (one that you DO want).

Read through all of the steps first before doing the exercise, as some steps will require you to do some preparation ahead of time:

THE STEPS:
1. **PRODUCE**
2. **DISRUPT**
3. **SWAP**
4. **PRAISE**
5. **REPEAT**

Write down the negative emotion you want to get rid of as it relates to doing or not doing something (e.g., When I think of exercising, I feel unmotivated.):

_____

_____

_____

1. **Produce it:** This is where you feel and experience the negative emotion you want to change. As soon as you feel the emotion or some physical symptoms of the emotion (heart racing, sadness, disgust, lull, procrastination), or anything at all, it's time to move on to the next step. Do not stay in the negative emotion for long.

2. **Disrupt it:** Break that pattern by loudly saying, "*ENOUGH*," and at the same time change your physical position. For example, if you are sitting, loudly say, "*ENOUGH*," and jump up to your feet. Changing your physical position (your physiology) is an important step to helping you change the emotion you are in that is not serving you well.

3. **Swap it**: In this step, you are going to generate an anchor. Anchoring is creating an association between a feeling and a touch or a sound. We create anchors all the time in our lives. For example, smelling a certain perfume may take you back to when you were a child watching your mother getting ready for work. Walking into a dentist's office and hearing the drill may send shivers of fear down your spine. A particular song may bring you happiness or sadness depending on what was transpiring in your life when you first heard it. Every time I hear the band, Air Supply (I know, I am completely dating myself right now), it takes me back to that care-free summer of when I was 11 and my family was renting a cottage with one of my best friends. We listened to Air Supply over and over that whole week as we were sunbathing and talking about life and boys.

I am sure you have heard about the experiment of Pavlov's dogs. Ivan Pavlov was a Russian scientist who was able to get the dogs to associate eating with the ringing of a bell. He would first ring the bell and then provide the dogs with food, and would notice the dogs salivating. After some time, he would only ring the bell, and the dogs would still salivate as if they were expecting food, even though no food was given. The dogs made an association (or anchor) with the ringing of the bell and food being brought to them, and thus would start salivating.

For the purposes of this exercise, you will want to associate (anchor) something that is positive and is the opposite of the emotion you want to replace. If you are procrastinating, you may want to become motivated; if you are frustrated, you may want to become calm; if you are sad, you may want to become happy. You can choose any positive emotion you want to achieve! Any positive feeling and behaviour is better than the negative feeling you want to get rid of.

Write down the positive emotion you would like to have instead:

_____

_____

_____

_____

_____

You will replace that negative emotion with the desired one you have chosen. When you interrupt the pattern of the negative emotion you have now, you will have a void that will need to be filled. You will fill this void with the new positive emotion. This step takes a little preparation ahead of time.

Look at the desired emotion you have chosen and recall a time when you were totally feeling that emotion. For example, if you want to change your procrastination to motivation, think back to a time when you felt super motivated, excited, and unstoppable! I want you to recall that time and feeling with a huge smile on your face and, as you do, I want you to lightly squeeze your right fist and say, "I've got it!" Make sure you are smiling the whole time during this process!!! When you smile, you change your physiology. You send positive chemicals throughout your body that make you feel good.

You are now anchoring feeling motivated and unstoppable to the squeezing of your fist and saying the words, "I've got it!" To add power and strength to your anchor, over the next 2–3 days as you go about your day, look for situations when you are feeling good; I mean really, really good! Cause yourself to feel good! Any time you catch yourself feeling good, excited, motivated, etc., put a big smile on your face, squeeze your right fist and say, "I've got it!" Do this over and over again for the next 2–3 days.

4. **Praise it:** In this step, you will reward yourself for doing such a great job! You can applaud yourself, pat yourself on the back, or

do a little dance. Make sure you are smiling during this process. Do whatever it takes to celebrate your achievement!

5. **Repeat it:** Repeat this exercise. The more you repeat it, the more you will realize that it becomes more and more difficult to get to that original undesired emotion and behaviour.

So here is the whole process; do the steps **quickly**:

- Sit down and recall the undesired feeling you want to change (e.g., unmotivated: make yourself feel bad, but don't stay in the feeling for long).

- Interrupt the pattern by saying the word, ENOUGH, and by jumping to your feet.

- Squeeze your fist and say, "I've got it!"

- Pat yourself on the back (or do your little dance).

- Repeat (sit back down and make yourself feel bad). Do this at least 10 times. Repeat these steps 10 times daily for 1 week.

You will find that you will no longer be able to feel that old emotion anymore, and at the very least, it will be much less intense than before.

My client, Jennifer T., implemented this to go from hating exercising to being motivated to exercise daily. Jennifer came to me to lose 20 pounds. She mentioned at the very first session how she hated any sort of physical activity. She found exercise boring and looked for any excuse possible not to do it. She would tell herself that she should go for a walk after dinner, and then she would proceed to check her emails, tidy up the house, and do any other activity except to go for that walk. Eventually, it would become dark outside and too late for her to go walking. Jennifer's behaviour was procrastination. She wanted to feel motivated when she thought about going for a walk because that would propel her to actually go for one.

I helped Jennifer apply the same process I outlined above. Before we went through the technique in the office, Jennifer was instructed to anchor the feelings of motivation and energy. Jennifer was coached to remember a time when she was super motivated and energetic. As she remembered that time, she would have to squeeze her right fist. She would then seek out times in the next couple of days when she felt energetic, motivated, and inspired. Each time, she would squeeze her right fist and say, "I've got it!"

During our next visit, Jennifer went through all of the steps:

1. *Produce it – that was easy. Jennifer started by sitting in the chair and recalling how she feels when she thinks of going for a walk. Just the thought of going for a walk would produce the feelings of doing something opposite—feeling uninspired and delaying the activity.*

2. *Disrupt it – She then jumped to her feet and said, "ENOUGH," and*

3. *Swap it: Jennifer squeezed her fist saying, "I've got it!"*

4. *Praise it: Jennifer would finish off this process by doing a silly dance.*

I instructed Jennifer to repeat this 10 times. On her 6th try, she reported that she could not even remember the old feeling of not being motivated, as it was now replaced with her feeling motivated and energetic. Jennifer's homework was to do this exercise every day until our next session. She called me 5 days later letting me know that she had been walking daily!

Here are some other examples of how you can use this exercise to help with feelings and behaviours you may want to change:

- Feeling annoyed with your children when they don't do their chores – you may want to replace this with feelings of calm.

- Feeling stressed while driving in traffic – you may want to replace this with feelings of being relaxed.

- Feeling anxious over a presentation – you may want to replace this with feelings of confidence.

- Feeling out of control when there is dessert in front of you – you may want replace this with feelings of being in control.

Focus on What You Want

Setting goals is extremely important in helping you achieve your outcomes. Your Unconscious Mind likes to keep things the way they are and that means keeping you from making changes. In an illogical way, this is the way in which it thinks it keeps you safe. Having a goal allows you to have direction and focus so that you can produce the results you want. Having a specific picture of a goal in mind activates your Private Investigator (the RAS) to search and bring to your attention all the important information which can help you achieve your results so it doesn't remain as background noise.

What is your reason for wanting to lose weight? Often, when I ask my clients this question, they say it is so they can be "happy." Now that's an interesting concept. Remember what I explained previously, that all of your feelings stem from your thoughts. This means that happiness is not something that can be attained from external factors (losing weight, having money, buying designer clothes) but is attained internally from your thoughts. How many times have you heard of people winning the lottery and not being any happier with their lives?

How many times have you heard of people attaining their goal weight and still being unhappy with themselves or their relationships? That is because happiness comes from within you. The reason you want to set goals is because, in the process, you get to overcome fears and barriers, and will become a better version of you, which has nothing to do with losing 50 pounds.

When you determine your goal, it is imperative that you write it down and keep it in a place where you can see it often. Make your goal as specific as possible and state it in the first person and present tense. This is where you state the "what" of the goal. Your goal may look something like this:

"I am celebrating my weight loss of 50 pounds on or before _____"
(Pick a date 6 months from today, including day, month, and year.)

You may find that as soon as you write that goal down, thoughts of failure, doubt, and judgment come up, and you start having negative thoughts of why you won't succeed. This is absolutely normal. In fact, if you have no negative thoughts, it might be because your goal is not big enough. A goal that takes you out of your comfort zone may produce negative thoughts. Your Unconscious Mind thinks of this as a threat to you; some big change is about to happen and your UM needs to keep you safe, even if keeping you safe is not serving you well. Pay attention to all the negative thoughts that come up, and write them down—all those thoughts that are trying to talk you out of striving for your goal.

Your list may look like this:

- I don't know if I can lose the weight.

- What's the point in trying this again? I've failed many times before.

- I won't have the time to organize my meals.

- I don't know how I will fit physical activity into my schedule.

- Maybe I'm just not meant to have a healthy body.

You are not going to ignore these thoughts and work against them. That will perpetuate that internal struggle between your conscious and unconscious desires and will not produce lasting results. I want you to float out into that date in the future where you have determined you will have accomplished your goal, and really feel, see, and hear what it is like to be so successful. What are you seeing? Feeling? Hearing? Is anyone giving you a congratulatory high five? Are you finally wearing the jeans you wanted to fit into? What are you saying to yourself? Are you saying, "I did it!" Remain in that future place of success and look back to now; address each and every negative thought you have. Remember that you determine the thoughts you have. You have a choice in what you think; it is completely in your power.

You will notice that when you do this exercise from the place of your future self, where your goal has already been accomplished, you will realize it is a very powerful place to be in. You just may realize that your negative thoughts and fears are almost silly. You will see that you have a lot of wisdom, insight, and power from that place. It is from that place that I want you to figure out the "HOW" of your goal. The neat thing in figuring out the "HOW" is working backwards from your future self to the present self.

Let's take the goal of losing 50 pounds in 6 months. Start from the place where your goal has already been accomplished and you have lost the weight. Now ask yourself, what was the last thing you had to do/learn to lose the last 10 pounds? Was it to learn about healthy cooking, or maybe increase the intensity of your physical activity? Write your answer down. Then ask yourself what you had to do to lose the 10 pounds before that? Write it down. And the 10 pounds before that? Write it down. Keep going back and determining what actions you had to take to reach each smaller goal until you go all the way to the first 10 pounds. What did you have to do to lose the first 10 pounds? Was it to become aware of your thoughts and how they relate to your feelings, which relates to your actions? Was it to start listening to your body when you are eating and following the hunger scale? For a free, print-ready download of a worksheet on goal setting, go to www.ItsNotAboutTheCheesecake.com.

You will see that by the end of this process, you will have the steps from your starting point (where you are now) and all the steps required along the way to reach your goal. Along the way, you may find that in this "HOW" process, there are aspects that you just don't know how to do. For example, you don't know how to read a food label and figure out what all the information means, or you don't know any recipes on how to cook vegetables, or you don't know how to plan your meals in advance. It is perfectly OK to not have the skills that may be required of you to get to your success. This is where you write down what is needed and ask yourself how you can obtain this skill or knowledge. Perhaps you need to find a coach to help you on your journey, or sign up for a cooking class, or make an appointment with a Registered Dietitian.

As you can see from the above example, the goal was broken down into 10-pound increments. Each 10-pound increment can then be further broken down into 5-pound increments, which can then be further broken down into 1-pound increments. If your goal is 1 year away, break it down into monthly goals; then, break those monthly goals into weekly goals, and then into daily goals. The smaller your goals, the easier it is to take action on them and have successes over and over. As you create a very specific picture of your goal, you are also revving up the RAS to scan your surroundings for you and bring to your attention all that is relevant to you achieving what you want— information that would have otherwise been deleted. All of a sudden, you may find that a friend tells you about a cooking class they are interested in attending and asks you if you want to join them. Or you find an awesome, healthy recipe in your email inbox, or you meet a person at your local coffee shop who ends up being a motivation and life coach. Your RAS is working for you to get you to your goal!

Limiting Beliefs Be Gone!

During my coaching sessions with clients, I use a number of modalities and tools to help uncover their unconscious limiting beliefs, clear them, and replace them with ones that will catapult them to success. I am going to teach you one exercise you can do to help clear your unconscious self-limiting beliefs and replace them with *empowering* ones! Read the exercise to the end before doing it. You can also record it and then play it back. Make sure you are sitting or lying comfortably with no distractions. Turn off any distraction such as your TV and phone, and ensure you are not driving.

Read the exercise slowly and softly.

Exercise:

Close your eyes and breathe deeply, in and out. Take a deep breath in, and slowly breathe out. Continue to take another 5 deep, slow breaths, in and out. Slowly and deeply. And just relax. Relax all the tension from your body. Continue breathing slowly and deeply. Relax your eyes. Relax your jaw. Relax your neck and shoulders. Continue to breathe in and out. Slowly and deeply. Let your mind completely relax. Your arms, your torso, and your legs are feeling heavy as you relax. You are feeling safe and warm as you relax. Concentrate on your breath as you slowly breathe in and out. In and out. Now, count slowly backwards from 10, as you continue to breathe. With each number, you will relax more and more. 10…..9…..8…..7….6…..5…..4…..3….2…..1 Breathing in and out, in and out.

I want you to visualize that you are lying in a hammock on the beach. Slowly swaying back and forth. The sun is keeping you safe and warm and you feel a slight breeze as you are swaying back and forth. You can smell the ocean and hear the birds chirping in the distance. Take in all the beauty of what is around you. All the sights and sounds.

Now, think about the goal you've identified that you would like to achieve (losing weight, fitting into your skinny jeans, getting control over your eating). Picture yourself trying to reach it and not succeeding. Failing at it once again. How does that look and feel, you not being able to lose the weight, or you regaining it all back? Having no control over your eating. Your pants feeling tight. How does that picture look? How does it feel being unsuccessful?

Continue breathing deeply. In and out. Far off in the distance, you notice another picture. It is much, much smaller. When you look at that picture, in it you see yourself achieving your goal. You are achieving the result you want. You are fitting into smaller clothes, you have reached your goal weight, you have complete control over what and how much you eat. You feel energized and motivated like you can achieve anything you set your mind to! As you continue to look, this picture is moving toward you and you are feeling more and more confident and empowered and motivated. It is getting stronger and stronger. You feel that you have all you need within you to achieve what you want. The picture is moving closer and closer. You feel you can achieve your goals. You are worthy to achieve what you want!

You are now seeing 2 pictures. The smaller, empowering one is at the top right corner and the other one is in front of you. Now, as quickly as you can, bring the smaller picture close and right in front of you, and send the picture you don't want off into the far distance. You must do this as quickly as you can say "switch." And go. Switch! Do it again. The picture you want in the right upper corner and the picture you don't want in front of you. And, "switch." The picture you don't want goes off into the distance. Do it again. "Switch." And again, "switch." Switch. Switch. Switch.

The picture of what you want is now firmly in front of you and is here to stay. When you think of being slim, of fitting into your jeans, of getting control over your eating, you see it all in front of you. You have an abundance of incredible, motivating, loving feeling! The picture of what you don't want is far off in the distance. The picture of what you DO want is coming even closer, and you step right into it and really look around with your own eyes, and see and embrace all the positive energy and feelings! It feels so incredible to achieve your results! Hear all the praise of friends and family around you of how proud they are of you!

Continue to breathe in and out. Come back into the room slowly, counting from 1 all the way up to 10. With each number you become more and more awake and energized. When you reach number 10, open your eyes, feeling exhilarated and motivated.

Repeat this exercise daily for 21 days.

Moving Forward

It is my hope that while reading this book, you actually went through and completed all of the exercises and techniques. Taking massive action will result in change! Reading the book and not going through the action steps will give you more awareness of why you haven't been successful in your weight loss efforts, but it will not result in any neurological change required to get you unstuck from where you are. It is my wish for you that you have been able to drop the self-criticism and self-judgment, and have replaced it with curiosity, compassion, and love. The answer to your success was never about the perfect diet or the right detox, or even your willpower; the answer was always inside of you. As a young child, you formed self-limiting beliefs about yourself, as well as patterns in using food for something other than physical hunger. Food provided a distraction, an avoidance, a comfort, and an inappropriate way to meet a deeper need.

You are now the Driver in your life, having full control of how you respond to any situation that comes your way! You have successfully squashed the power of the Mean Girl and have directed your personal private detective (RAS) to work for you in bringing your attention and focus to what is important in achieving your goal. All the information you have previously deleted is now available to you. Continue to use the techniques as you move forward toward your goals and desires. Remember that you have the power for great change. If you have not yet completed the action steps, go to www.ItsNotAboutThe Cheesecake.com and download the free bonus worksheets NOW!

About the Author

Sulana Perelman's passion is to help women struggling with yo-yo dieting and emotional eating. Having been a yo-yo dieter for most of her life and overcoming her own weight struggles, Sulana has made it her mission to lead as many women as possible to their road of success.

Sulana completed a Degree in Food and Nutrition at Ryerson Polytechnic University, as well as a Master's of Health Science in Community Nutrition at the University of Toronto. She is a Master Coach in Neuro-Linguistic Programming, Time Line Therapy ™ and a Trainer in Hypnosis. Sulana uses a variety of unique and holistic modalities in her private coaching practice and offers Weight Loss Breakthrough Programs to her clients.

Sulana lives with her family in Toronto, Canada. You may reach Sulana at sulana@sulanaperelman.com

Notes

Notes

Notes

Notes

Notes

Notes

Notes

www.ingramcontent.com/pod-product-compliance
Lightning Source LLC
Chambersburg PA
CBHW071136280326
41935CB00010B/1250